CONTENTS

Introduction

Pellet grills have always appealed to both professional and amateur BBQers – and for good reasons. They are convenient, easy to operate, and capable of producing classic barbecue meals.

Pellet grills have been around for nearly forty years. And during that time, they have evolved from being a creative wood-and-charcoal smoker alternative to becoming a multi-purpose cooker that can roast, smoke, sear, and also bake.

The origins of wood pellet grills (also known as pellet smokers) can be traced to the 1970's oil crisis and the ensuing demand for an alternative fuel source. Wood pellets, one of the widely accepted oil alternatives, are small eraser-sized hardwood capsules made of compressed sawdust. A decade after the crisis, the Traeger's Oregon-based heating company, previously known to produce Pellet stoves, became famous for its innovative Pellet grill.

Joe Traeger, along with aviation engineer Jerry Whitfield, started experimenting for a pellet-burning furnace in 1982, developed a prototype in 1985, obtained a patent in 1986, and began manufacturing the first models of the Traeger Wood Pellet Grills and Smoker in 1988. For 20 years, the Traeger company owned the sole rights to produce wood pellet grills. During this time, the cooking appliance gained a massive following of barbecue enthusiasts.

Traeger Wood Pellet Grills & Smoker Cookbook will explain the basic components and operation of the grill. It will also reveal some delicious recipes you can recreate with the multi-purpose grill. Proceed to Chapter 1 to know more.

Chapter 1: Essentials of Trager Wood Pellet Grill

What is Traeger Wood Pellet Grill?

Traeger Wood Pellet Grills are electric grills that use wood pellets as their fuel source. The specially designed wood pellets can also be used as flavor enhancers to give food an excellent smoky taste. With his grill, Joe Traeger revolutionized barbecuing and made it convenient and straightforward. Traeger Wood Pellet Grill and Smoker does not require constant monitoring and can be left to regulate itself while cooking.

There are five methods of cooking with the grill; they include:

▢ Indirect grilling
▢ Direct grilling
▢ Smoking
▢ Roasting
▢ Baking

Despite fierce competition, Traeger grills continue to be the world's No 1 best-selling wood pellet grill because of its mastery of the wood-fired cooking craft. The grill is capable of transforming a simple fare into an extraordinary dish with its wood-fired flavoring. The grill temperatures can range from 150°F to well over 375°F to enable it to grill, sear, roast, smoke, and bake. It produces consistent results.

Components of Wood Pellet Grill and their Functions

There are five models of Traeger Pellet Grills available, depending on the size and capabilities. The models include:

- Pro Series
- Ironwood Series
- Timberline Series
- Portable Grill Series
- Commercial Grill Series

Some of the components featured in the models are:

Pellet Hopper: This is the part of the grill that stores the wood pellets. It's recommended to keep it filled to prevent interruption of cooking activities. The amount of pellets used depends on the time and temperature required for cooking a particular meal.

Porcelain-Coated Grill Grate: This holds the food to be prepared. It is coated with porcelain to prevent the sticking of meals. The grate is also very easy to clean.

Cast Iron Grate: This grate allows for even distribution of heat when grilling. It creates a perfect sear when used.

Steel Construction: Made from cold-rolled steels, they are durable and reliable as a cover for the Traeger grill. It helps with the regulation of temperature and can be cleaned easily because of its non-stick surface.

Convection Blower: This is important to the grill as it is responsible for maintaining a constant flow of air to keep the pellets in the Firepot aflame.

Auger: This conveys the pellets from the hopper to the Firepot.

Auto Start Firepot: This is where the wood pellets are ignited for cooking. It is controlled by the Thermostat and does not require any external firing methods.

Hot Rod Ignitor: When turned on, it causes the pellets in the Firepot to ignite and rise to the temperature selected on the Thermostat Controller.

Fire Baffle Plate: It is positioned around the Firepot and serves as a deflector shield to retain heat. The plate ensures that the heat produced is absorbed and spread evenly to the cooking grates.

Thermostat Controller: This is used to set the temperature of the wood pellet grill. It controls the Hot Rod Ignitor and ensures that the selected temperature is maintained throughout cooking.

Grease Drain Pan and Bucket: Used during indirect grilling, baking, roasting, and smoking. The Grease Drain Pan collects the grease produced during cooking and transports it to the Grease Bucket through the Grease Drain Tube.

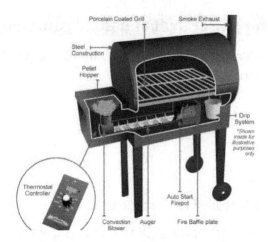

Smoke Exhaust: This is used to control the flow of air out of the grill. It is essential for maintaining the temperature of the cooking chamber.

Step-by-Step Operation of the Traeger Grill

The grill is designed to be easy to operate and use. After purchasing a Traeger Wood Pellet Grill & Smoker, the first step is to assemble the cooking appliance. Instructions for the assemble is present in the accompanying Owner's Manual. Once assembled, acquaint yourself with some of the components itemized above.

Here is a quick step-by-step instruction on how to start a fire in the Wood Pellet Grill:

1. **Open the Steel Door** and remove the following components from the grill: porcelain grill grate, the heat baffle, and grease drain pan.
2. **Ensure the Grill Switch is in the "O" position (OFF).** Then connect the power cord to a suitable electrical outlet.
3. **Switch ON the grill ("|" position) and turn the thermostat controller to Smoke.** Check if the Auger is rotating. You will be able to notice the rotation of the Auger through the pellet hopper. Also, place your hand over the Firepot to feel the movement of the convection blower. The Hot Rod should start to turn red.
4. **Fill the hopper with specially designed Traeger Barbecue Pellets** and turn the thermostat controller to High. Wait a few minutes for the pellets to travel from the hopper to the Firepot.
5. **Switch the thermostat controller to Smoke** and allow the wood pellet flames in the Firepot to rise. Then, switch the thermostat controller to the Shutdown cycle to cool down the grill.
6. **Reset the components** (porcelain grill grate, the heat baffle, and grease drain pan) of the grill to their proper position. Line the drain pan with heavy-duty aluminum foil for easy cleaning.
7. **Ensure the Steel Door remains open, then switch the thermostat controller to Smoke**. When pellets will start to produce whitish-gray smoke, close the door and set the thermostat controller to the desired setting/temperature.
8. **Season the grill when cooking for the first time** by setting the Thermostat to High and running for 45 minutes with the steel door closed.
9. **Always preheat grill at the desired temperature for 10 minutes** before placing food on grates.

Traeger Wood Pellet Grill vs. Gas or Charcoal Grills

The three types of grills are all capable of cooking meat, but they have different modes of operation. When compared with the other grills, Traeger Wood Pellet Grill & Smoker is superior because of the following reasons:

- **Taste:** Traeger Grill infuses a woody and smoky taste into the meals prepared on it, unlike when gas or charcoal is used. The combined moist, smoky, and woody taste is far superior.
- **Ease:** Of the three types, the wood pellet grill is more comfortable to operate and use. The Traeger grill trademark slang "Set it & Forget it" draws its meaning from the fact that all you have to do is fill the hopper and set the desired cooking temperature.

Convenience: The Traeger Grill has an app that can connect to the grill via Wi-Fi. The technology is called WiFIRE, and it allows you to control your grill with your smartphone. Traeger Wood Pellet Grill enables you to change the temperature while sitting on your couch, unlike charcoal or gas grills that require manual adjustment.

Tips and Tricks of Using a Traeger Grill

While the Traeger Wood Pellet Grill is easy to use, some people do have issues with it due to inexperience. The following tips will help you start on the right foot:

- **Store your pellets properly**. Pellets go bad when exposed to humid environments. Wet wood pellets do not ignite when set aflame, and they may cause extensive damage to the Auger when used. Store them in a close-lid container to prevent contact with moisture.
- **Wrap thermocouple with aluminum foil to prevent grease build-up**. When the thermocouple is covered in grease, it is unable to read temperatures accurately. Alternatively, you can clean thermocouple after every use.
- **Cover the grill when not in use**. The Traeger grill is an electrical appliance and is susceptible to water damage. Cover grill with weatherproof vinyl covers or keep in shades when idle.
- **Clean grill regularly.** Develop a schedule for cleaning your grill to prevent damage or fire accidents.
- **Try out new recipes and utilize every function.** There are two types of Traeger grill users; the passive users that barbeques once every three months, and the enthusiasts that discover new ways to cook with their beloved grill. Traeger Wood Pellet Grill is versatile and can cook different types of dishes, whether Reverse Seared Tri-tip or Spaghetti Squash. Try to find new and exciting ways to make your favorite dishes on the grill.

Cleaning and Maintenance of your Traeger Grill

When pellets are burned, they produce organic vapors and tar that combine with water to form creosote. These creosotes are highly flammable and can lead to unpredictable fire hazards. To protect yourself from fire accidents and other unpleasant effects of using a dirty Wood Pellet Grill, you need to clean the grill periodically (or after every meal if possible).

Here are some places you need to clean to reduce the risk of fire:

1. Clean the Smoke Exhaust with warm, soapy water or biodegradable degreaser. Scrape accumulated creosote with a wooden or any other non-metallic tool.
2. Inspect the Grease Drain, Grease Drain Tube, and Grease Bucket for grease build-up. Clean regularly with soapy water and a soft brush or wipe with paper towels and rags. Lining grease Bucket with aluminum foil will make clean-up easier.
3. Clean Steel construction with warm, soapy water and rags to remove grease. Do not use abrasive materials to scrub or it will peel off the non-stick surface.
4. Clean Porcelain grill while after every meal, while **warm.** Do this with a long-handled cleaning brush to prevent burns and injuries.
5. Remove ash accumulated inside and around Firepot. Sweep ash with a whisk broom or metal fireplace shovel.

NB: These activities should be performed when the grill is COLD and disconnected from a power source, except stated otherwise, to prevent burns and electrical accidents.

Frequently Asked Questions

⧄ Why Won't My Wood Pellet Grill Ignite?

Ensure the Grill is connected correctly to a power source, then start the ignition process again. If this does not work, disconnect the grill and uninstall the Thermostat Controller. Check for a blown fuse and any other possible error. Reinstall thermostat and plug the grill to check if Convection Blower and Auger are functioning correctly. At this point, if you're unable to detect the reason for the ignition failure, replace Hot Rods or contact your Local Traeger dealer for support.

⧄ Why are The Wood Pellets Not Delivered to the Firepot?

Pellets take about 7-10 minutes to travel from the hopper to the Firepot. If the pellets do not arrive at the Firepot after this time, switch off the grill and disconnect from the power source. Reinstall the Auger and Draft Inducer Fan (small fan at the back of the auger motor). Then, reconnect and switch on the grill. If the Auger motor does not work and the fan is rotating, contact your local Traeger dealer to replace the Auger. If both systems are working but the Auger is still not delivering wood pellets, replace the digital counter.

⧄ What Temperature Do I Use with My Thermostat Controller When Cookbook Recipes require Smoke, Medium, and High?

When cooking Non-Traeger designed recipes, you may find it challenging to convert the required cooking temperatures to fit the Traeger Grill. Here is a brief conversion table for the temperature to set your thermostat when Smoke, Medium, or High settings are mentioned or vice versa.

Requested Smoker Control Settings	Suggested Thermostat Settings
Smoke	150-180°F (also smoke on Traeger Grill)
Medium	225-275°F
High	350-400°F

Chapter 2: Grilling Recipes

Bearnaise Sauce with Marinated London Broil

Béarnaise sauce is a classic sauce, and it tastes incredibly delicious when dribbled on London Broil.

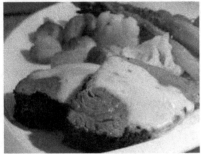

Prep time and Cooking Time: 50 minutes with an overnight marinade

Ingredients To Use:

- 2 cups of Rory's marinade
- 1-1/2 cups of béarnaise sauce
- 2-1/2 pound of London broil

Step-by-Step Directions:

1. Place London broil in a big baking dish, pour marinade over the steak, then refrigerate it over the night.
2. Set the grill for direct cooking at 300°F. Use maple pellets for a robust woody taste.
3. Remove London broil from the marinade the following morning. Place it on the preheated grill and cook for 15 minutes before flipping and grilling the other side for 10 minutes. Serve immediately with béarnaise sauce.

Nutritional value per serving:

Calories: 367g, Fat: 39g, Carbs: 53g, Protein: 32g

Grilled Eggplant with Pine Nuts

Eggplant has many functions; one of them is that it boosts liver function. It also helps the body to release trapped heat. The combination of eggplant and pine nuts helps to cool the body system. It tastes especially delicious when prepared on a grill with wood as fuel.

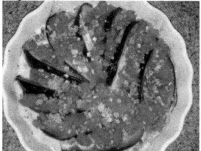

Prep time and Cooking Time: 20 minutes | Serves: 8

Ingredients To Use:

- 1/3 cup of fresh lemon juice
- 1/4 cup of pine nuts
- 2 medium of eggplants
- 2 cloves of garlic
- 3 Tbsp of fresh parsley, chopped
- 2 tomatoes
- 1-1/2 tsp of salt
- Squares of flatbread
- Freshly ground black pepper to taste
- 1/2 cup of olive oil
- 1/4 cup of chopped scallion

Step-by-Step Directions:

1. Set the grill for direct cooking at 250°F. Use cherry wood pellets for a sweet fruity flavor.
2. Perforate eggplants with a fork and place it on hot cooking grates. Flip periodically to ensure both sides are grilled. Do this for 10 minutes.
3. Wrap scorched eggplants in aluminum foil and place them on the cooking grids. Cook until eggplants become soft.
4. Pierce tomatoes with a skewer and arrange on the grates. Grill until skin wrinkles.
5. Peel off the scorched skin of the eggplants and put them in a bowl. Add the grilled tomatoes to the bowl and mash together with a fork
6. To the bowl containing the mashed eggplant and tomato, add the pepper, salt, pine nuts, lemon juice, oil, and garlic. Mix ingredients thoroughly.
7. Sprinkle scallions and parsley over the mixture. Serve it immediately with flatbread.

Nutritional value per serving:

Calories:67kcal, Carbs:9g, Fat:4g, Protein: 1g

Veal Kidney on Skewer

Veal kidneys are incredibly delicious when adequately seasoned and grilled. Treat yourself to this rare delicacy on your Traeger grill.

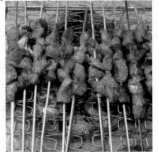

Prep time and Cooking Time: 30 minutes | Serves: 4

Ingredients To Use:

- Salt with ground pepper, preferably fresh
- 8 slices of bacon
- Bearnaise Sauce
- 2 veal of kidney, fat removed
- 2 Tbsp of peanuts or vegetable oil

Step-by-step Direction to Cook:

1. Set the grill for direct cooking at 300°F. Use hickory wood pellets to give scallions a robust taste.
2. Dice kidney to obtain about 46 pieces. Also, cut the bacon into 2-inch pieces
3. Arrange kidney and bacon on a skewer. Prepare as many shewer as possible with the materials available, then brush the skewers with oil.
4. Carefully arrange the skewers on the preheated grill and let it cook for about 10 minutes. Flip, season with salt and pepper on it, then cook for another 10 minutes.
5. Serve immediately with béarnaise sauce if available.

Nutritional value per serving:

Calories: 233.4kcal, Fat: 38g, Carbs: 39g, Protein: 22.3g

Lamb Burger Spiced with Curry

Have you ever tried to use lamb meat to make a burger pattie? If not, you're missing out on the incredibly unique and flavorful taste the meat gives the burger. Try it now on your Traeger wood pellet grill.

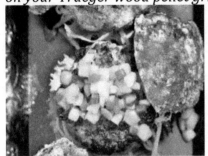

Prep time and Cooking Time: 20 minutes | Serves: 4

Ingredients To Use:

- 1/2 tsp of turmeric
- 1 tsp of ground coriander
- 1 fresh chili should be seeded and minced, preferably jalapenos chili
- 1 tsp of ground cumin
- 1-1/2 pound of boneless lamb, preferably shoulder.
- Salt and black pepper, shredded carrot
- Red onion with scallion
- Red ball pepper, diced mango

Step-by-Step Directions::

1. Set the grill for direct cooking at 300°F. Use maple pellets for a spicy, smoky taste.
2. Pulse the lamb and onions in a food processor and obtain a coarse texture.
3. Add the cumin, jalapenos chili, pepper, coriander, salt, and turmeric to a bowl. Mix thoroughly, then add the blended lamb. Stir gently.
4. Form 4 patties with the lamb mixture.
5. Grill lamb patties for 10 minutes, then flip and grill the other side for another 10 minutes
6. Serve immediately with mango, onion, and shredded carrot.

Nutritional value per serving:

Calories: 200kcal, Protein: 19g, Fat: 15.5g, Carbs:0g.

Grilled Clam with Lemon-Cayenne Butter

This is an easy clam recipe. There's no better way to cook clam than to grill it.

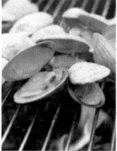

Prep time and Cooking Time: 15 minutes | Serves: 2

Ingredients that will use:

- 2 tsp of lemon juice, preferably fresh
- Large pinch of salt (kosher)
- 2 dozen of littleneck clams
- 1 large clove of garlic
- Chives, freshly chopped
- 4 Tbsp of unsalted butter, already melted
- Pinch of cayenne pepper

Step-by-Step Directions::

1. Set the grill for direct cooking at 300°F. Use alder wood pellets for mild taste and aroma.
2. Mash garlic and salt with a mortar and pestle to form a paste.
3. Scoop the paste into a small bowl and add cayenne pepper, butter, and lemon.
4. Grill clam over the preheated cooking grid for 5 minutes. When clam is ready, it will open. Carefully transfer opened clam to the bowl containing lemon-cayenne butter. Do not spill the clam-juice when transporting.
5. Gently mix the clam and butter until it is well-combined.
6. Serve immediately with chives.

Nutritional value per serving:

Calories: 148kcal, Carbs: 31g, Fat: 19g, Protein: 25g

Grilled Flank Steak

There are several ways to make a flank steak; by grilling, roasting, smoking, braising, etc. For this recipe, the grilling method is applied.

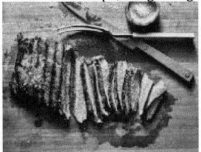

Prep time and Cooking Time: 2 hours 15 minutes | Serves: 6

Ingredients To Use:

- 1/2 cup of soy sauce
- 1-1/2 pound of flank steak.
- 1/2 cup of bourbon
- 1/2 cup of water

Step-by-Step Directions::

1. Set the grill for direct cooking at 300°F. Use hickory wood pellets for a strong taste and aroma.
2. Pour the soy sauce, 1/2 cup of water, and bourbon in a bowl. Whisk together to make a marinade. Pour the marinade inside a food storage bag and add the steak to the bag. Keep in the refrigerator for 2 hours to allow flavors to combine and penetrate steak.
3. Remove from the refrigerator and dry with a paper towel.
4. Grill the steak for about 30 minutes, flipping every five minutes to ensure both sides are equally cooked.
5. Cover the steak with foil paper and allow it to rest for about 5 minutes.
6. Serve.

Nutritional value per serving:

Calories: 370kcal, Carbs: 45g, Protein: 25.5g, Fat: 32 g.

Ginger and Chili Grilled Shrimp

Grilling brings out the best taste and flavor in shrimps. Ginger is an excellent ingredient for infusing the shrimps with aroma and taste.

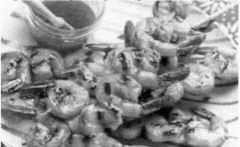

Prep time and Cooking Time: 1 hour 15 minutes | Serves: 6

Ingredients To Use:

- 1 tsp of salt, kosher
- 2 mangos, riped, peeled, and chopped
- 1 Tbsp of fresh ginger, grated
- 2 cloves of garlic, crushed
- 1-1/4 pound of jumbo shrimp, deveined and peeled.
- 2 jalapenos, chopped
- 1/2 cup of buttermilk, low-fat
- 1/2 tsp of black pepper, ground
- 1 lime, small and also cut into wedges (6)

Step-by-Step Directions:

1. Set the grill for direct cooking at 150°F. Use hickory wood pellets for a robust taste.
2. Pour the ginger into a bowl, add buttermilk, jalapenos, garlic, pepper, and salt. Mix thoroughly.
3. Put shrimps inside the same bowl, and mix well with a wooden spoon. Allow it to marinate in the refrigerator for an hour
4. Arrange 2 mango chops, 3 shrimps on a water-soaked wooden skewer. Do this for the other 5 skewers.
5. Place shrimp skewers on the grates and grill for 10 minutes, or until the shrimps turn opaque. Serve immediately with the lime wedge

Nutritional value per serving:

Calories: 80kcal, Protein: 20g, Fat:1.3g, Carb: 1.2g

Grilled Scallion Salad

Scallion has a mild taste and can be grilled or smoked. The combination of all the ingredients in this recipe results in a delicious meal.

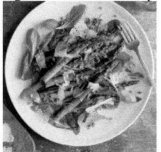

Preparation and Cooking Time: 20 minutes | Serves: 4-6

Ingredients To Use:

- 1/3 cup of rice vinegar
- 2 tsp of sugar
- 1 Tbsp of sesame oil
- 1 Tbsp of gochugaru
- 1 pound of scallion, untrimmed
- 1 Tbsp of sesame seeds

Step-by-Step Directions:

1. Set the grill for indirect cooking at 250°F. Use hickory wood pellets to give scallions a robust taste.
2. Brush sesame oil on scallions, then arrange it on the cooking grid. Grill with for about 8 minutes.
3. Remove scallions from heat and rub with sugar, vinegar, sesame seeds, and vinegar. Serve immediately.

Nutritional value per serving:

Calories: 56kcal, Carbs: 13g, Fat: 7g, Protein: -g

Grilled Chili Burger

The perfect burger recipe for the 4th of July! Try this spicy burger for a vibrant Traeger grill experience.

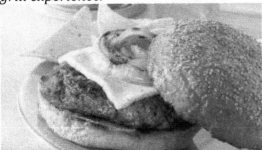

Prep time and Cooking Time: 20 minutes | Serves: 8

Ingredients To Use:

- 1 tsp of chili powder
- 4 tsp of butter
- 2 pounds of round steak, twice-grounded
- 1 clove of garlic
- Salt and ground pepper, preferably freshly ground
- 1/4 cup of bread crumbs

Step-by-Step Directions::

1. Set the grill for direct cooking at 300°F. Use maple pellets for a robust and woody taste.
2. Pour the meat inside a bowl and add the rest of the ingredients. Mix until well-combined. Mold the meat mixture to form 8 patties.
3. Arrange patties on the preheated cooking grid and grill for 10 minutes before flipping and grilling the other side for another 10 minutes.
4. Serve immediately with hamburger buns.

Nutritional value per serving:

Calories: 260kcal, Protein: 13g, Fat: 10.5g, Carbs: 29.9g.

Seafood on Skewers

There are different kinds of seafood and there are many recipes used in making them. Swordfish is the seafood we will be talking about.

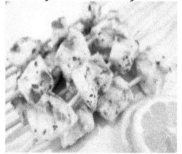

Prep time and Cooking Time: 40 minutes | Serves: 4

Ingredients To Use:

- 2 Tbsp of peanuts or corn oil
- 16 cubes of swordfish
- 8 sea scallops, big
- Salt and ground pepper, fresh
- 16 cubes of monkfish
- 12 jumbo shrimp
- Sauce Bearnaise

Step-by-Step Directions:

1. Set the grill for direct cooking at 200°F. Use oak wood pellets for rich, woody taste.
2. Arrange four pieces of alternating swordfish and monkfish pieces, shrimps, and scallops on a metal skewer. Repeat this for the other three skewers. Rub oil on the skewers.
3. Place the skewers on the preheated grill, and cook for 10 minutes. Flip to the other side and season with salt and pepper. Allow the other side to cook for another 10 minutes. Serve it with béarnaise sauce.

Nutritional value per serving:

Calories: 82kcal, Protein: 20.5g, Fat: 15g, Carb: 16g

Beef Tartare Burger

Burgers have never tasted better! With your Traeger grill, you can prepare your beef pattie with an additional woody taste.

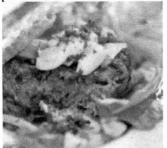

Prep time and Cooking Time: 30 minutes | Serves: 4

Ingredient To Use:

- 1 Tbsp of capers
- 1 shallot, already peeled
- Salt with pepper
- 1 medium of clove garlic
- 1-1/2 pound of fatty chuck
- 2 anchovy fillets, optional
- 1 medium-cooked egg, chopped
- 2 tsp of Worcestershire sauce
- 1/2 cup of parsley, preferably freshly chopped
- 1/2 tsp of tabasco sauce
- White onion and peeled lemon slices

Step-by-Step Directions:

1. Set the grill for direct cooking at 300°F. Use maple pellets for a strong, woody taste.
2. Pour garlic, beef, anchovies, shallot, and capers inside a food processor. Pulse until it is has a coarse texture (soother than chopped, but not by much).
3. Mix the parsley, Worcestershire sauce, salt, pepper, and tabasco in a bowl. Stir together with blended beef. Mold the mixture to form 4 patties.
4. Grill the meat for about 3-4 minutes (rare). Flip and grill until the other side is done.
5. Serve immediately with caper, onion, parsley with egg, lemon.

Nutritional value per serving:

Calories: 216kcal, Protein: 20g, Fat: 16g, Carbs: 45g

Grilled Tuna Burger with Ginger Mayonnaise

It's difficult to blend fish and form it into a pattie without a form of glue (egg or fat). This recipe replaces the need for glue by using grilled tuna as a burger pattie.

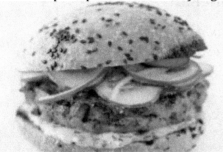

Prep time and Cooking Time: 20 minutes | Serves: 4

Ingredients To Use:

- 1 Tbsp of sesame oil, optional
- 4 Tbsp of ginger, optional
- 4 hamburger buns
- Black pepper, freshly ground
- 2 Tbsp and 1 tsp of soy sauce
- 4 of 5 ounces of tuna steak
- Natural oil
- 1/2 cup of mayonnaise

Step-by-Step Directions:

1. Set the grill for direct cooking at 300°F. Use maple pellets for a robust woody taste.
2. Rub soy sauce on the tuna steak and season with pepper.
3. In another bowl, prepare a rub by mixing the ginger, mayonnaise, 1 tsp of soy sauce, and sesame oil.
4. With a brush, apply the rub on the tuna steak then grill for 10 minutes before flipping. Grill the other side for another 10 minutes.
5. Serve immediately with fish between buns. Add mayonnaise and ginger as layers.

Nutritional value per serving:

Calories: 220kcal, Protein: 21.5g, Fat: 16g, Carbs: 23g.

Chapter 3: Roasting Recipes

Lemon And Thyme roasted with Bistro Chicken

Everyone has a simple chicken roast recipe, and for good reasons: a well-roasted chicken requires little adornment. This simple recipe uses lemon, butter, salt, and thyme as seasonings.

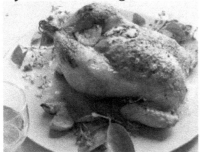

Prep time and Cooking Time: 25 hours | Serves: 4

Ingredients To Use:

- 1 4pounds chicken
- 3 Tbsp of unsalted butter, melted
- 1 lemon
- 1 Tbsp of thyme, fresh and chopped.
- Salt and ground black pepper, to taste

Step-by-Step Directions:

1. Season chicken with salt and pepper as desired. Make sure to rub seasoning all over, including the inner cavities. Refrigerate seasoned chicken, uncovered, for 24 hours.
2. Preheat the grill for direct cooking at 420°F (*High*). Use mesquite wood pellets for a distinctive, strong woody taste.
3. Put the lemon zest, chopped thyme, and butter in a bowl, then mix. Rub the mixture all over the chicken, and put half lemon in the chicken.
4. Place the chicken in a roasting pan and roast for about 35 minutes. Turn it to the other side and roast for 15 minutes or until internal temperature reads 160°F.
5. Cool for 10 minutes before slicing and serving.

Nutritional value per serving:

Calories: 388.9kcal, Protein: 41.8g, Carbs: 73.4g, Fat: 52g.

Curried Chicken Roast with Tarragon and Custard

This is a perfect recipe for birthdays, graduations, and other celebrations. The taste of the chicken produced is ethereal – crisp, juicy, and tender.

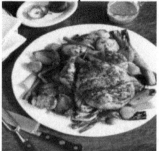

Prep time and Cooking Time: 1 hour 45 minutes, | Serves: 4

Ingredients To Use:

- 3 Tbsp of olive oil
- 1 Tbsp of salt, kosher
- 1 4pounds chicken
- 1/2 cup of grain mustard, whole
- 3 Tbsp of tarragon, freshly chopped
- 1 tsp of black pepper, freshly ground
- 1 Tbsp of curry powder

Step-by-Step Directions::

1. Preheat the grill for direct cooking at 420°F (*High*). Use hickory wood pellets for a robust taste.
2. Mix the salt, olive oil, mustard, tarragon, pepper, and curry powder in a bowl. Coat the prepared rub all over the chicken with a grill brush. Put the chicken inside a Ziploc bag and refrigerate for an hour.
3. Roast the chicken on the preheated grill for 35 minutes. With a tong, flip the chicken and roast for another 15 minutes, or until the internal temperature of the thigh reads between 168-169°F.
4. Allow cooling for about 10 minutes before slicing and serving.

Nutritional value per serving:

Calories: 330kcal, Protein: 34.1g, Carbs: 48g, Fat: 39g

Rosemary Chicken Glazed with Balsamic with Bacon Pearl Onions

Pearl onions are difficult to roast correctly, but they taste delicious when cooked with chicken and other types of meat.

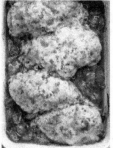

Prep time and Cooking Time: 50 minutes | Serves:4

Ingredients To Use:

- 2 Tbsp of unsalted butter
- 1 Tbsp of brown sugar, light
- 1 4pounds chicken
- 2 Tbsp of balsamic vinegar
- 1/4 pound of bacon
- 1 Tbsp of thyme, fresh
- 3/4 of pearl onions, frozen

Step-by-Step Directions::

1. Rub black pepper and salt all over the chicken, including cavities. Put the chicken on a rack and keep inside the refrigerator for 24 hours.
2. Preheat the grill for direct cooking at 420°F (*High*). Use mesquite wood pellets for a distinctive, strong woody taste.
3. Mix the vinegar, butter, brown sugar, and thyme in a bowl, then rub it on the chicken with a brush.
4. Put the pearl onion, balsamic mixture, and bacon under the chicken in the roasting pan.
5. Roast the chicken on the preheated grill for 35 minutes. Flip the chicken with a tong and roast for another 15 minutes, or until the internal temperature of the thigh reads 165-170°F.
6. Rest for 5 minutes, then serve the chicken with the bacon and the onion.

Nutritional value per serving:

Calories: 390kcal, Protein: 39g, Fat: 48g, Carbs: 53.

Roast Chicken with Caramelized Shallots and Fingerling Potatoes

Fingerling potatoes also called tiny tubers, are great are for pan-fried or roasted meals.

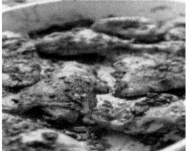

Prep time and Cooking Time: 50 minutes | Serves: 4

Ingredients To Use:

- 4 peeled shallots
- 2 Tbsp of unsalted butter
- 1-1/2 of fingerling potatoes
- 1 Tbsp of sherry vinegar
- 1 of 4 pounds of chicken
- 2 Tbsp of rosemary, fresh
- Kosher salt and black pepper

Step-by-Step Directions::

1. Rub black pepper and salt all over the chicken, including cavities. Put the chicken on a rack and keep inside the refrigerator for 24 hours. However, if the chicken has been brined, you can skip this step and move on to the roasting.
2. Preheat the grill for direct cooking at 420°F (*High*). Use maple wood pellets for a strong, woody taste.
3. Mix the butter, and 1 Tbsp of rosemary inside a bowl. Rub the mixture all over the chicken. In another bowl, mix the pepper, rosemary, potato, and shallots. Pour the mixture into the roasting pan and place the chicken on it.
4. Roast the chicken on the preheated grill for 35 minutes. Flip the chicken and roast for another 15 minutes, or until the internal temperature of the thigh reads between 165-170°F.
5. Serve after cooling for 10 minutes.

Nutritional value per serving:

Calories: 256kcal, Fat: 24g, Protein: 32g, Carbs: 46g

Roast Bison Sirloin

This recipe involves the use of a low-temperature roasting method. The temperature is ideal for grass-fed bison.

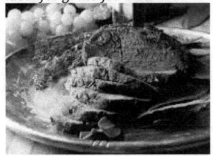

Prep time and cooking book: 3 hours | Serves: 7

Ingredients To Use:

- 3 Tbsp of spice rub
- 1 6pounds bison sirloin roast, boneless
- 2 Tbsp of herbs, either fennel or thyme or sage or rosemary
- 3 Tbsp of olive oil

Step-by-Step Directions::

1. Remove roast from refrigerator and allow to thaw until temperature reads between 50-55 °F.
2. Preheat the grill for indirect cooking at 200°F. Use alder wood pellets.
3. Rub the surface of the meat with oil, then season with salt and pepper. Place bison in a skillet and Place on the cooking grid. Add the herbs and spices rub.
4. Roast for about 2 ½ hours or until internal temperature reads 120-125°F.
5. After removing the roast from the oven, allow it to rest for 15 minutes before carving and serving.

Nutritional value per serving:

Calories: 140kcal, Protein:29g, Carbs:0g, Fat: 3g.

Roasted Tri-Tip with Spanish Adobo Rub

An excellent meal to prepare on the weekends when everyone is home. It's easy to make on the Traeger Grill; just put the meat in the oven and relax on your couch with a beer.

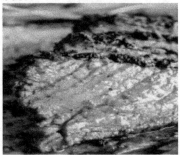

Prep time and Cooking Time: 2 hours 45 minutes | Serves: 5

Ingredients To Use:

- 1 Tbsp of olive oil
- 2 tsp of salt
- 3 cloves of garlic, already peeled
- 1 tsp of black pepper
- 2 tsp of marjoram, preferably freshly chopped
- 3 Tbsp of paprika, Spanish
- 1/4 cup of vinegar, sherry
- 1 of 2pound of tri-tip roast

Step-by-Step Directions::

1. Preheat the grill for direct grilling at 420°F (*High*). Use hickory wood pellets for a robust woody taste.
2. Prepare the rub by pulsing garlic, paprika, marjoram, and vinegar in a food processor. Rub the mixture produced all over the meat. Allow meat to marinate for 2 hours.
3. Place the meat on the cooking grid and sear for 2 minutes per side.
4. Reduce the temperature of the grill to 350°F and roast the meat for 45 minutes or until the internal temperature reads 140- 145°F.
5. Allow to rest for 10 minutes before serving.

Nutritional value per serving:

Calories: 373.5kcal, Protein: 34.5g, Carbs: 49g, Fat: 38.3g

Mushroom with Fennel Dressed with Roasted Chicken

Fennel and mushroom dressing is excellent with roast chicken. The meal is also healthy and delicious.

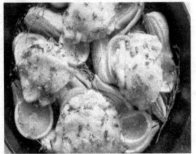

Prep time and Cooking Time: 22 hours 50 minutes | Serves: 4

Ingredients To Use:

- 8 sun-dried tomatoes, oil-packed
- 4pound chicken
- Salt with black pepper
- 1-1/2 Tbsp of thyme
- 10 ounces of mushroom, preferably white button
- 1/2 pound of crusty bread
- 4 cloves of garlic, preferably smashed
- 1 Tbsp of balsamic vinegar
- 2 Tbsp of butter without salt.
- 1 fennel bulb

Step-by-Step Directions::

1. Rub black pepper and salt all over the chicken, including cavities. Keep in the refrigerator for 22 hours.
2. Remove chicken from the refrigerator and rub with butter. In a big bowl, mix sun-dried tomato, mushroom, fennel, garlic, thyme, salt, and pepper. Then put the mixture into the roasting pan along with the chicken.
3. Roast the chicken on the preheated grill for 35 minutes. Flip the chicken with a tong and roast for another 15 minutes, or until the internal temperature of the thigh reads between 165-170°F.

Nutritional value per serving:

Calories: 290kcal, Carbs: 35g, Fat: 42g, Protein: 38g

Roasted Steak

This recipe works with all types of beef. When cooked with garlic, roasted steak is low in calories and carbs.

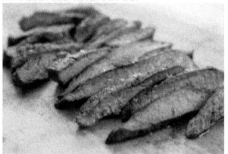

Prep time and Cooking Time: 12 hours 30 minutes | Serves: 5

Ingredients To Use:

- 2 Tbsp of rosemary, preferably freshly chopped
- 2 tsp of salt
- 1 Tbsp of thyme, preferably fresh leaves
- 1/2 cup of olive oil
- 1-1/2 tsp of black pepper
- 1 of 3-inch steak
- 5 cloves of garlic, preferably thinly sliced

Step-to-step Direction to Cook It:

1. Make the marinade by cooking garlic until it is soft, then add rosemary and thyme. Cook for about 1 minute.
2. Rub black pepper and salt all over the steak, then put it inside a Ziploc bag with the garlic mixture. Keep in the refrigerator overnight.
3. Remove steak from the refrigerator the next morning, and discard the garlic marinade. Roast the steak on the preheated grill for 30 minutes or until the internal temperature reads 160°F.
4. Serve the steak and season with salt and black pepper before eating.

Nutritional value per serving:

Calories: 334.5g, Carbs: 42g, Fat: 35g Protein: 32.5g,

Rib Roast and Yorkshire Pudding with Bacon and Rosemary Jus

This type of food is usually cooked during Thanksgiving because it is delicious to share. Thyme and garlic are part of the main ingredients.

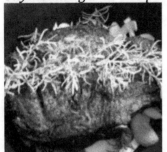

Prep time and Cooking Time: 45 minutes | Serves: 10

Ingredients To Use:

- 1 Tbsp of black pepper
- 1 bacon with rosemary jus
- 3 Tbsp of thyme, preferably fresh leaves
- 6 cloves of garlic, already peeled
- 2-1/2 Tbsp of salt
- 2-1/2 Tbsp of olive oil
- 1 of 5-bone of rib-eye roast, standing
- 1 scallion with parmesan Yorkshire pudding

Step-by-Step Directions::

1. Put garlic inside a running food processor. Scrape it into a bowl, mix with pepper, salt, thyme, and oil until a paste is formed.
2. Preheat the grill for direct cooking at 350°F. Use mesquite wood pellets for a distinctive, strong woody taste.
3. Press the herb mixture into the sliced ribs. Put the ribs in the roasting pan and roast both sides for 20 minutes or until internal temperature reads 145°F.
4. Allow the ribs to rest for 10 minutes before serving. After then, serve with Yorkshire pudding.

Nutritional value per serving:

Calories: 250kcal, Protein: 25.6g, Carbs: 33g, Fat: 25.5g.

Sandwich with Roasted Beef

For a restaurant-worthy roasted beef sandwich, try this recipe on your Traeger Wood Pellet Grill & Smoker.

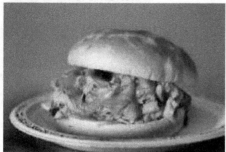

Prep time and Cooking Time: 25 minutes | Serves: 4

Ingredients To Use:

- Butter
- Barbecue sauce
- 1 pound of beef roast
- 4 hamburger buns

Step-by-Step Directions:

1. Set the grill for direct cooking at 300°F. Use hickory pellets.
2. Roast the beef on the grill for 20 minutes or until internal temperature reads 135°F.
3. Lightly rub butter on the hamburger buns, then arrange the roasted beef between the buttered buns. You can also put the barbecue sauce well on the meat.
4. Serve immediately.

Nutritional value per serving:

Calories: 340kcal, Protein: 22g, Fat:12.9g, Carb: 32.9g.

Pork Rack Roasted with Romesco Sauce in Spanish-Style

It is a Spanish-style family meal. This method of roasting pork is one of the best, mostly because already brined pork is used, and brining takes 1-2 days.

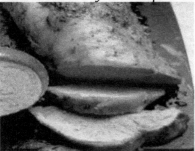

Prep time and Cooking Time: 85 minutes |Serves: 6

Ingredients To Use:

- 2 Tbsp of olive oil
- 4 piquillo pepper, whole
- 2 Tbsp of minced garlic
- 1 Tbsp of salt
- 1 Tbsp of paprika, Spanish
- 1 cup of spanish sherry, dry
- 2 tsp of black pepper, dried
- 1 of 7-bone of pork rib loin roast
- 1/4 cup of olive oil
- 1/4 cup of bread crumb
- 6 cloves of already sliced garlic
- 1 Tbsp of marjoram
- 1/2 cup of almond, roasted
- 2 tsp of garlic, minced
- 1 peeled Roma tomato, halved and seeded

Step-by-Step Directions:

1. Preheat the grill for direct cooking at 300°F. Use maple wood pellets.
2. Mix all the ingredients in a small bowl, then brush it over the pork roast. Place the pork roast in the roasting pan and roast for about 15 minutes.
3. Get a baking dish and pour the garlic, pepper, tomato, oil in it. Put the pork inside it and roast for another 30 minutes. Check if it is done to your taste. If not, keep roasting until you are satisfied.
4. Remove roast from cooking grid and allow to rest.
5. Separate the oil in the roasting pan, then add the tomato, roasted pepper, sherry, and already processed almond from the food processor. Mix until it forms a paste. Add season with pepper and salt.
6. Serve the pork with the prepared sauce.

Nutritional value per serving:

Calories: 280kcal, Protein: 32g, Fat: 40g, Carbs: 49.9g

Sweet Potato Spiced Fries

French fries taste incredibly good when roasted with a wood pellet grill. Try it out with this simple recipe.

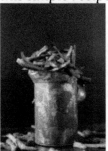

Prep time and Cooking Time: 30 minutes | Serves: 4

Ingredients To Use:

- 1 tsp of kosher salt
- 2 Tbsp of olive oil
- 1 tsp of paprika
- 1/2 tsp of cumin, ground
- 2 pounds of sliced sweet potatoes
- 1 tsp of brown sugar, light
- 1 tsp of chili powder
- 1 tsp of garlic powder

Step-by-Step Directions:

1. Mix the brown sugar, paprika, garlic powder, chili powder, salt, and cumin in a bowl.
2. Mix the sliced potatoes and oil in a separate bowl, then add the brown sugar mixture and toss well. Pour the coated potatoes into a roasting pan and roast until it is brown and tender. This will take about 15-20 minutes.
3. Serve as soon as possible.

Nutritional value per serving:

Calories: 177.85kcal, Protein: 23.9g, Carbs: 21.9g, Fat: 39.8g.

Chapter 3: Smoking Recipes

Smoked Chicken with Perfect Poultry Rub

The perfect poultry rub helps smoked chicken taste better. It comes in different colors and can either be in paste form or dry.

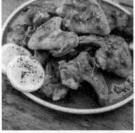

Prep time and Cooking Time: 3 hours 15 minutes. Serves: 2

Ingredients To Use:

- 2 Tbsp of onion, powder
- 1/4 cup of black pepper, freshly ground
- 2 Tbsp of dry mustard
- 3/4 cup of paprika
- 4pound chicken
- 3 lemon
- 2 tsp of cayenne
- 1/4 cup of sugar
- 1/4 cup of celery salt

Step-by-Step Directions:

1. In a bowl, mix the onion powder, paprika, black pepper, dry mustard, cayenne, sugar, celery, salt, and 2 lemons.
2. Add your chicken to the rub and slice some parts so that the ingredients will find their way in.
3. Preheat the grill for 15 minutes at 225°F. Use apple wood pellets for a distinctive, strong woody taste.
4. Place the coated chicken on the preheated grill and smoke for 3 hours or until internal temperature reads 160°F.
5. Allow chicken to cool, then serve.

Nutritional value per serving:

Calories: 255kcal, Protein: 35g, Carbs: 42g, Fat: 35g.

Seafaring Seafood Rub with Smoked Swordfish

The swordfish in this recipe can be replaced with any type of seafood, such as shrimps, swordfish, or stripe bass.

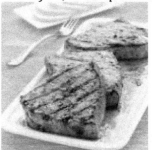

Prep time and Cooking Time: 2 hours 15 minutes | Serves: 6-8

Ingredients To Use:

● 4 tsp of garlic, ground
● 2 tsp of paprika
● 1 tsp of nutmeg, ground
● 1/2 tsp of allspice, ground
● 4 tsp of ginger, ground
● 1 tsp of cayenne
● 2 Tbsp of celery seed
● 1/4 cup of sea salt
● 4 tsp of black pepper, freshly ground
● 2 pounds of swordfish
● 2 tsp of brown sugar

Step-by-step Directions to Cook it:

1. Preheat the grill for 15 minutes at 225°F. Use oak wood pellets for a distinctive, strong woody taste.
2. Combine all the ingredients (except swordfish) in a bowl. Mix thoroughly.
3. Add the swordfish to the bowl and gently coat it with the mixture. Do not allow the swordfish to break.
4. Place the coated swordfish directly on the preheated grate and smoke for 2 hours or until fish turns opaque and flakes.
5. Serve immediately.

Nutritional value per serving:

Calories: 173kcal, Carbs: 27g, Protein: 21.9g, Fat:19g.

Sweet Sensation Pork Meat

Pork rack is succulent, and it can be grilled, roasted, or smoked. Smoking helps to reduce the fat content.

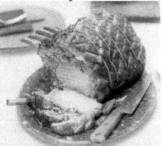

Prep time and Cooking Time: 3 hours | Serves: 3

Ingredients To Use:

- 2 tsp of nutmeg, ground
- 1/4 cup of allspice
- 2 tsp of thyme, dried
- 1/4 cup of brown sugar
- 2 pounds of pork
- 2 tsp of cinnamon, ground
- 2 Tbsp of salt, kosher or sea

Step-by-Step Directions:

1. Preheat the grill for 15 minutes at 225°F. Use hickory wood pellets
2. Combine all the ingredients (except pork) in a bowl. Mix thoroughly.
3. Slice the sides of the pork meat in 4-5 places. Put some of the ingredients into the slices and rub the rest over the pork.
4. Place the pork on the preheated grill and smoke for 3 hours or until internal temperature reads 145°F.
5. Allow it to rest before serving.

Nutritional value per serving:

Calories: 300kcal, Protein: 36g, Carbs: 45g, Fat: 31g

Slum Dunk Brisket

Smoking a brisket is unique; temperature control is very important because of the length of time it takes to finish. With your Traeger grill, all you have to do is set the temperature and forget it.

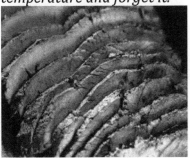

Prep time and Cooking Time: 9 hours of smoking, 20 minutes prep. Serves: 9

Ingredients To Use:

- 1/4 cup of pickle juice, dill
- kosher or sea salt
- barbecue sauce
- 1/4 cup of mustard, Dijon
- 6 pounds of brisket
- 6 strips of bacon, artisanal
- Black pepper

Step-by-Step Directions::

1. Preheat the grill for 15 minutes at 250°F. Use apple wood pellets for a distinctive, strong woody taste.
2. Mix the pickle juice and mustard in a bowl. Trim off the fats on the brisket, then rub the mustard mixture on it—season with salt and pepper. Put bacon on the brisket.
3. Place the coated brisket and bacon directly on the grates, close the steel construction, and smoke for 9 hours or until internal temperature reads 160°F.
4. Remove the brisket from the grill when it ready. Allow it to rest for an hour before carving and slicing.

Nutritional value per serving:

Calories: 355.3kcal, Fat: 47.2g, Protein: 30.9g, Carbs: 41g

Smoked Beef Tenderloin

This is another recipe that requires temperature regulation when cooking. The combination of beef tenderloin with horseradish sauce is perfect.

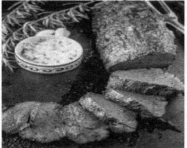

Prep time and Cooking Time: 3 hours | Serves: 8

Ingredients To Use:

- Black pepper, freshly ground
- Vegetable oil
- 4 pound of beef tenderloin
- Kosher or sea salt
- 2 Tbsp of olive oil
- Horseradish sauce

Step-by-Step Directions::

1. Preheat the grill for 15 minutes at 250°F. Use cherry wood pellets.
2. Season tenderloin with salt and black pepper. Place it on the baking sheet and brush all the sides of the tenderloin with olive oil.
3. Place the tenderloin in the preheated grill and smoke for 3 hours or until internal temperature reads 160°F.
4. Remove from grill when it is done and allow it to rest for 10 minutes.
5. Serve the tenderloin.

Nutritional value per serving:

Calories: 325kcal, Fat: 44.9g, Protein: 33.8g, Carbs: 50g.

Cherry Smoked Strip Steak

Smoking strip steak takes about 2 hours. Doing it on a Traeger grill results in a moist, smoky, delicious piece of meat.

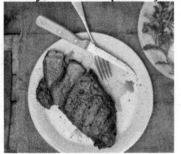

Prep time and Cooking Time: 70 minutes. Serves: 3

Ingredients To Use:

● Kosher or sea salt
● Olive oil
● Black pepper
● 1-1/2 pound of rib steak

Step-by-Step Directions::

1. Preheat the grill for 15 minutes at 225°F. Use maple wood pellets.
2. Season the steak with salt and black pepper.
3. Place the seasoned steak directly on the grates and smoke for 2 hours or until internal temperature reads 160°F.
4. After smoking, rub olive oil on the steak then return it to the grates of the grill. Increase the temperature to 300°F and grill it for another 10 minutes.
5. Serve it hot.

Nutritional value per serving:

Calories: 289.5kcal, Protein: 35.9g, Fat: 40.5g, Carbs: 51g

Smoked Pork Shoulder

Adding onion powder to pork produces a good flavor. Garlic, cayenne pepper, black pepper, and salt are the main ingredients of this recipe.

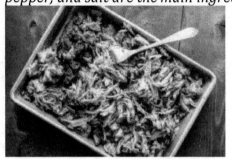

Prep time and smoking time: 7 hours 40 minutes. Serves: 8

Ingredients To Use:

- 2 tsp of garlic powder
- 4 tsp of salt, either sea and kosher
- 2 tsp of onion powder
- 4 tsp of black pepper
- 2 tsp of garlic
- 6 pounds of pork shoulder
- 1 tsp of cayenne pepper
- Carolina vinegar sauce
- 11 sesame seed buns, already split
- 3 Tbsp of melted butter.

Step-by-Step Directions::

1. Preheat the grill for 15 minutes at 245°F. Use apple wood pellets for a distinctive, strong woody taste.
2. Mix onion powder, pepper, garlic powder, cayenne, salt, and black pepper in a bowl. Use your fingers to rub the mixture on the meat.
3. Place the pork shoulder inside the grill and smoke for 7 hours.
4. Slice the pork, and the bones will remove effortlessly.
5. Put the shredded pork in a plate, add sauce and stir it together
6. Serve it with butter and toasted buns.

Nutritional value per serving:

Calories: 203kcal, Fat: 25g, Carbs: 30g, Protein: 16g

Honey Cured Ham Ribs

Smoking ham rib takes about 4-6 hours. The combination of honey and curing salt gives the ham rib a pleasant taste

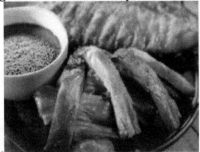

Prep time and Cooking Time: 3 days 5 hours 20 minutes. Serves: 3

Ingredients To Use:

- 3/4 cup of honey
- 1-1/2 cup of cold water
- 1-1/2 cup of hot water
- 8 cloves
- 1 rack of spareribs
- 3/4 cup of kosher or sea salt
- 1-1/2 tsp of pink curing salt
- 3 bay leaves
- Mustard seed caviar

Step-by-Step Directions:

1. Place the ribs on the baking sheet. Mix the hot water, honey, coarse salt, and pink curing salt until the salt and honey dissolve in the water. Allow it to cool to room temperature.
2. Add the rib to the cooled brine and transfer it to a Ziploc bag. Keep in the refrigerator for 3 days.
3. Remove the ribs from the refrigerator and place it on the baking pan.
4. Preheat the grill for 15 minutes at 250°F. Use pecan wood pellets for a spicy, nutty taste.
5. Put the ribs on the grates of the grid and smoke for about 4 hours.
6. Serve immediately with mustard seed caviar.

Nutritional value per serving:

Calories: 375kcal, Protein: 45g, Fat: 43.5g, Carbs: 55g

Monster Smoked Pork Chops

This simple recipe does not need many ingredients, except if you desire additional flavor. Black pepper, sugar, kosher salt, curing salt, vegetable oil are the most important ingredients

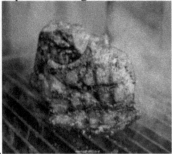

Prep time and Cooking Time: 2 hours 30 minutes, 12 hours for brining. Serves: 4

Ingredients To Use:

- 1/3 cup of sugar
- 4 tsp of pink curing salt
- Vegetable oil
- 1 cup of kosher or sea salt
- 1-1/4 pound pork chops
- 1/4 hot water
- 1/4 cold water

Step-by-Step Directions::

1. Put the pork on a big baking pan. Mix the salt, curing salt, sugar, and hot water in a bowl. Add the pork to the mixture, and refrigerate for 12 hours.
2. Preheat the grill for 15 minutes at 250°F. Use pecan wood pellets
3. Bring the pork out and remove the brine from the pork.
4. Smoke the pork for about two and a half hours until it is done or until the internal temperature reads 145°F.
5. Brush olive oil all over the sides of the pork. Then increase the temperature of the cooker to 300°F and grill the pork chop for another 5 minutes until it is done.

Nutritional value per serving:

Calories: 350kcal, Protein: 35g, Carbs: 45g, Fat: 40g.

Smoked Irish Bacon

The unique flavor of Irish bacon is obtained from smoking, and this takes about 2 hours 30 minutes

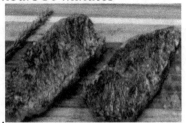

Prep time and Cooking Time: 3 hours | Serves: 7

Ingredients To Use:

- 1 bay leaf
- 2/4 cup of water
- 2/3 cup of sugar
- 6 star anise, whole
- 1 cup of fresh fennel, preferably bulb and fronds
- 2 spring thyme, fresh
- 1 clove of garlic
- 2 tsp of curing salt
- 2-1/2 pound of pork loin
- 1-1/2 tsp of peppercorns, black
- 1-1/2 tsp of fennel seed

Step-by-Step Directions:

1. In a big stockpot, mix the fennel seeds, peppercorn, star anise, and pork roast for about 3 minutes. Also, mix the sugar, water, thyme, garlic, curing salt, coarse salt, and bay leaves in a pot and, boil for 3 minutes until the salt and sugar dissolves.
2. Place the pork loin in a Ziploc bag, seal it, and put it in a roasting pan. Keep refrigerated for 4 days.
3. Preheat the grill for 15 minutes at 250°F. Use pecan wood pellets.
4. Remove the pork from the brine and place on the grates of the grill. Smoke it for 2 hours 30 minutes or until internal temperature reads 145°F.
5. Serves immediately or when it is cool.

Nutritional value per serving:

Calories: 309kcal, Fat: .7g, Protein: 30.6g, Carbs: 40g

Mutton Barbecued and Black Dip

A castrated lamb or a lamb that does not produce wool anymore is used to make this meal. Smoking takes about 7 hours.

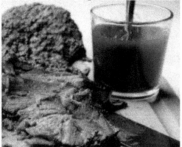

Prep time and Cooking Time: 7 hours 20 minutes. Serves:7

Ingredients To Use:

- Kosher or sea salt
- 7 hamburger buns
- 2 Tbsp of butter
- Sliced dill pickle
- 6 pounds of lamb shoulder
- Black dip

Step-by-Step Directions:

1. Season lamb with salt and pepper
2. Preheat the grill for 15 minutes at 250°F. Use pecan wood pellets.
3. Put the lamb inside black dip, then transfer it to the smoking rack. Smoke the lamb for 7 hours.
4. Put the already smoked lamb on a dish or board. Allow it to rest for 10 minutes. Remove the fat lumps.
5. Put butter on the buns, pile the lamb on the buns, and add pickle slices.
6. Serve it with black dip.

Nutritional value per serving:

Calories: 279.9kcal, Fat: 30.2g, Protein: 35g, Carbs: 49g

Lamb Shanks, Smoke-Braised

Smoking of this lamb shank can be done in an open space or closed environment. Smoking takes about 5 hours.

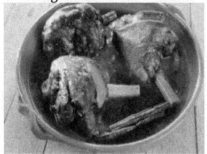

Prep time and Cooking Time: 5 hours 20 minutes | Serves: 2

Ingredients To Use:

- 1/2 cup of brown sugar
- 2 cups of water
- 4 strips of orange
- 2 cinnamon sticks
- 3 whole of star anise
- 1/2 cup of soy sauce
- 2 shank of lamb
- 1/2 cup of rice wine
- 3 Tbsp of sesame oil, Asian

Step-by-step Directions:

1. Put the lamb shank on an aluminum foil paper.
2. In a bowl, mix the sesame oil, water, soy sauce, and brown sugar in a bowl until the sugar dissolves. Add the cinnamon stick, orange zest, and star anise to the bowl. Pour the mixture on the lamb.
3. Preheat the grill for 15 minutes at 250°F. Use alder wood pellets
4. Place the lamb shank on the cooking grates with the foil. Smoke the lamb for 5 hours, until it is brown.
5. Remove the lamb from the smoker and place it on a board to trim off excess fat. Serve immediately.

Nutritional value per serving:

Calories: 255kcal, Carbs: 46g, Fat: 36g, Protein: 34.1g.

Chapter 5: Braising Recipes

Buttered Green Peas

Buttered and tendered green beans are excellent for Thanksgiving as a side dish for beef roast and shrimps.

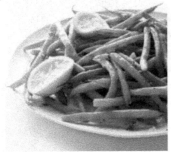

Prep Time and Cooking time: 30 minutes | Serves: 1-2

Ingredients To Use:

- 1/2 cup butter, melted
- Kosher salt
- 24 oz green beans, trimmed
- 1/4 cup veggie rub

Step-by-Step Directions:

1. Preheat the wood pellet smoker-grill to 345°F using pellets of your choice
2. Pour the beans into a baking pan lined with parchment sheets and rub melted butter over the beans. Season with salt. Place the baking pan on the cooking grid.
3. Arrange the beans on the pan with a tong and pour the veggie rub over it.
4. Braise the beans until tender and lightly browned. Flip after 20 minutes.
5. Serve.

Nutritional value per servings:

Calories: 93kcal, Carbs: 9.5g, Fat: 3.8g, Protein: 3.8g

Beer-Braised Pork Shank

Pork shank slowly braised with beer, and spicy sauce satisfies cravings for delicious comfort food and is best served with puréed potatoes.

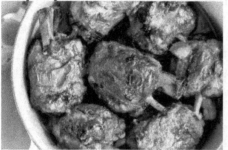

Prep Time and Cooking Time: 23 minutes |Serves:6

Ingredients To Use:

- 2 Tbsp Flour
- Kosher salt
- Ground black pepper
- 2 Tbsp olive oil
- 2 Tbsp butter
- 1 medium onion, diced
- 2 carrots, trimmed and diced
- 1 Tbsp garlic, minced
- 1 cup dried mushrooms
- 2 cup beef broth
- 2 Tsp chili powder
- 2 thyme sprigs
- 2 Tsp coffee, instant
- 1 Tbsp Worcestershire sauce
- 12 oz dark beer, porter
- 2 dried bay leaves

Step-by-Step Directions:

1. Preheat wood pellet smoker-grill to 300^0F with the cover of the grill closed for 10 minutes.
2. Hold pork shank together with a butcher string and sprinkle pepper and salt over it.
3. Place a Dutch oven on the cooking grid. Add oil and pork shanks. Cook shank until brown on both sides.
4. Remove shanks from heat and transfer to a plate.
5. Sauté onions, carrots, and garlic in Dutch oven until tender, about 8 minutes.

6. Mix in beef broth, beer, and Worcestershire sauce to the sautéed vegetables. Increase the temperature and bring to boil. Allow simmering at *Medium* temperature until one-third of the liquid is gone.
7. Add tomato paste, coffee, thyme, chili powder, and bay leaves.
8. Transfer pork shanks from the plate into the Dutch oven and scoop sauce atop it.
9. Cook shanks until tender, about 3 hours.
10. Combine in a bowl, butter, and flour. Add the flour mixture in the last hour to thicken the sauce.
11. Take out bay leaves and thyme springs. Cut out butcher's string. Serve pork shank with gravy atop it and garnish with parsley.

Nutritional value per servings:

Calories: 85kcal, Carbs: 2.0g, Fat: 3.5g, Protein: 7.0g

Beef Pot Roast

This warm dinner recipe makes a complete savory meal that's well suited for slow cooking with little effort.

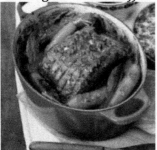

Prep Time and Cooking time: 3 hours 10 minutes | Serves: 6

Ingredients To Use:

- 3 cup beef stock
- 1 cup carrots, chopped
- 1 Tbsp garlic, minced
- 1/4 cup softened butter
- 1 Tsp ground black pepper
- 2 red onions, chopped
- 4lb chuck roast
- 1 Tbsp kosher salt
- 1Tbsp sage, chopped
- 1/2 cup red wine

Step-by-Step Directions:

1. Preheat Traeger Grill & Smoker to 300^{0}F with the cover of the grill closed for 10 minutes.
2. In a stockpot, put in red wine, beef stock, butter, garlic, carrot, red onion, sage, and chuck roast—season with pepper and salt. Stir the contents and cover the pot.
3. Transfer stockpot to the preheated grill; close the grill lid and leave to cook for 3 hours, until the roast reaches an internal temperature of 203^{0}F.
4. Serve.

Nutritional value per servings:

Calories: 487kcal, Carbs: 19g, Fat: 17g, Protein: 6.0g

Butter-Braised Springs Onions with Lots of Chives

Spring onions with caramelized butter sauce have a soft, pleasant taste. This recipe can also be used as a side dish.

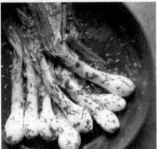

Prep Time and Cooking Time: 25minutes|Serves:3

Ingredients To Use:

- 1lb spring onions, trimmed
- Kosher salt
- 1/4 tsp chives, chopped
- 4 Tbsp unsalted butter

Step-by-Step Directions:

1. In a large skillet, add onions, 1/2 cup water, two tablespoons butter and sprinkle in the salt. Cover skillet and bring to a boil. Reduce heat and simmer onion until almost tender, about 15 minutes. Remove cover, stir continuously and leave onions to cook for another 5 minutes, until fork-tender.
2. Take out onions and place them on a plate. Heat the liquid in skillet until it reduces to about two teaspoons, then add the remaining butter. Transfer onions to the skillet and stir it in with the sauce. Garnish with chives.

Nutritional value per servings:

Calories: 129kcal, Carbs: 4.0g, Fat: 12g, Protein: 2.0g

Rosemary Braised Lamb Shank

Lamb shanks cooked to tender perfection, slowly simmered in rosemary and red wine sauce is a family favorite dinner delight.

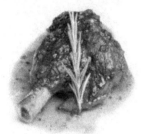

Prep Time and Cooking Time: 2 hours 45 minutes | Serves:4

Ingredients To Use:

- 2 spring's rosemary
- 2 celery stalk
- 3 garlic clove, minced
- 2 cups red wine
- 2 carrots, diced
- 4 lamb shanks, fat trimmed
- 2 Tbsp olive oil
- 2 Tbsp chophouse steak
- 2 onion, diced

Step-by-Step Directions:

1. Preheat wood pellet smoker-grill to 350^0F.
2. Brush oil over lamb shanks, arrange on grill and grill on each side until brown, about 2 minutes.
3. Transfer the shanks from grill to a heatproof baking pan; add onions, carrots, garlic, onions, rosemary springs, beef stock, red wine, and Chophouse steaks.
4. Reduce grill temperature to 325^0F
5. Cover baking pan with aluminum foil and place on grill.
6. Braise the shanks for 2-1/2 hours on smoker-grill, until tender.

Nutritional value per servings:

Calories: 254kcal, Carbs: 27 g, Fat: 1g, Protein: 6g

Korean BBQ Short Ribs

Ribs cut along the bone and marinated for at least 6 hours before braising is an exquisite homemade flavorful dish.

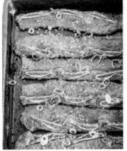

Prep Time and Cooking Time: 5 hours 40 minutes | Serves:4

Ingredients To Use:

- 1 cup beef broth
- 1 Tsp ginger, minced
- 1/2 cup of soy sauce
- 1 Tsp toasted sesame seeds
- 6 beef short ribs, membrane removed
- 2 Tbsp brown sugar
- 1 Tbsp beef rub
- 2 garlic cloves, minced
- 1 Tbsp sriracha sauce

Step-by-Step Directions:

1. Preheat wood pellet smoker-grill to 250°F.
2. Combine in a medium bowl, brown sugar, garlic, ginger, beef broth, soy sauce, sriracha, sesame, beef, and brisket rub, and then set aside.
3. Place ribs in a baking dish and add the marinade. Cover and leave to marinate in a refrigerator for about 6-12hours.
4. Transfer marinated short rib to the top of the grill grate. Grill for 4 hours; rub leftover marinade juice on the rib occasionally.
5. Remove rib from the grill and leave to rest on a platter for 15minutes. Serve.

Nutritional value per servings:

Calories: 662kcal, Carbs: 17g, Fat: 85g, Protein: 35g

Red Wine Braised Short Ribs

Braising short ribs in wine sauce gives it a dark color and a rich burst of flavor. The beef easily slides off the bone and melts in your mouth.

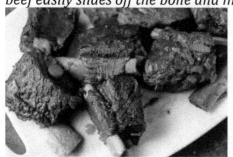

Prep Time and Cooking Time: 9 hours | Serves: 12

Ingredients To Use:

- Kosher salt
- 1/2 cup onion, thinly sliced
- 4 garlic cloves, smashed
- 5lb brisket, flat-cut
- 2 Tbsp olive oil
- 2 bay leaves
- 6 spring's thyme
- 28 oz of canned whole tomatoes
- 4 medium carrots cut lengthwise
- 750ml red wine
- 1 Tbsp tomato paste

Step-by-Step Directions:

1. Preheat wood pellet smoker-grill to 350^0F.
2. Place brisket on a flat surface and sprinkle pepper and salt on it.
3. Pour oil into a large ovenproof pot and cook the brisket in it for about 10 minutes or until meat browns. Remove brisket and place on a plate, then discard fat in the pot.
4. Add onions, garlic, thyme, bay leaves, tomatoes, wine, tomato paste, celery, salt, and pepper in a large pot. Return brisket to pot, fat side up, and then cover the pot. Braise brisket on the grill for about 3hours, until fork tender.
5. Place carrot on brisket, then cook until carrot is tender and braising liquid in the pot is concentrated. It will take about 30 minutes.
6. Remove fat from the sauce—transfer brisket and braising liquid to a bowl. Cover and leave to rest for at least 4 hours.
7. When ready to serve, preheat grill to 325^0F. Heat braising liquid and brisket for about 1 hour.

Nutritional value per servings:

Calories: 459kcal, Carbs: 8g, Fat: 25g, Protein: 34g

Pork Carnitas

Carnitas, know as "little meats," are perfect for tacos, burritos, and sandwiches. This recipe is also easy to make.

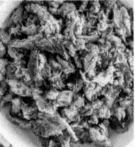

Prep Time and Cooking Time: 3 hours | Serves: 6

Ingredients To Use:

- Lime wedges
- 3 jalapeno pepper, minced
- A handful of cilantro, chopped
- 1 cup of chicken broth
- 2 Tbsp olive oil
- Corn tortilla
- 3lb pork shoulder, cut into cubes
- Queso Fresco, crumbled
- 2 Tbsp pork rubs

Step-by-Step Directions:

1. Preheat wood pellet smoker-grill to 300^0F.
2. Mop the rub over the pork shoulder. Place pork shoulder in a cast-iron Dutch oven and pour in chicken broth. Transfer pot to grill grate and cook 2½ hours, until fork tender.
3. Remove the cover, bring to a boil then reduce the liquid in pot by half. All this happens within 15 minutes.
4. Place a tablespoon of bacon fat on the skillet and fry the pork for about 10 minutes, until crisp.
5. Take out pork and serve with cilantro, jalapeno, lime, queso fresco, and corn tortillas.

Nutritional value per servings:

Calories: 254kcal, Carbs: 6g, Fat: 6g, Protein: 41g

Belgian Ale-Braised Brisket

This combination of Belgian style beer and flat cut juicy brisket is perfect for a winter supper.

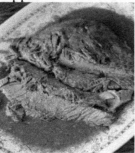

Prep Time and Cooking Time: 3 hours | Serves: 6

Ingredients To Use:

- 1/4 cup Dijon mustard
- 2 bay leaves
- 1/4 cup all-purpose flour
- 1/4 cup dark brown sugar, packed
- 2 Tbsp bacon fat
- 2 medium onion, thinly sliced
- Kosher salt
- 4lb beef brisket, flat cut, untrimmed
- 1 Tbsp grated ginger
- 4 cups beef broth
- 750ml bottle Belgian style tripel ale

Step-by-Step Directions:

1. Preheat wood pellet smoker-grill to 400°F.
2. Rub brisket in salt and leave in a reusable plastic bag for 8 hours at room temperature.
3. In a small bowl, mix ginger, brown sugar, and ginger.
4. Remove brisket from the bag, rub mustard over brisket, and place on the grill grate. Roast for 40 minutes, until the top, is brown.
5. Transfer brisket to a plate and set aside.
6. Reduce the temperature of the grill to 300°F.
7. Heat bacon fat in a cast-iron Dutch oven placed on the grill. Add onions and sprinkle in the salt. Stir continuously and cook until brown, about 10 minutes.
8. Reduce heat and stir in flour and cook for another 4 minutes. Add ale, bay leaves, and stock, and then allow to simmer. Put in brisket and cover the lid of the Dutch oven.
9. Braise brisket for 4 hours with the grill cover closed.

10. Remove bay leaves and place brisket on a platter. Allow resting of brisket for 20 minutes before carving.
11. Serve brisket with braising liquid.

Nutritional value per servings:

Calories: 387kcal, Carbs: 35g, Fat: 21g, Protein: 14g

Bourbon Braised Beef Short Ribs

Short ribs braised I n a mixture of Worcestershire sauce, bourbon, soy sauce, mustard, and beef stock until amazingly tender is a perfect warm dish.

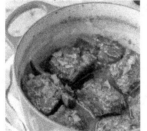

Prep Time and Cooking Time: 3 hours 15 minutes | Serves:6

Ingredients To Use:

- 2 Tbsp Worcestershire sauce
- 3 Tbsp soy sauce
- 2 Tbsp bourbon
- 1/2 cup Dijon mustard
- 1 cup beef stock
- 12 beef short ribs

Step-by-Step Directions:

1. Preheat wood pellet smoker-grill to 250^0F, with the lid closed for about 15 minutes
2. Mix the Worcestershire sauce, mustard, and molasses.
3. Brush sauce on each side of the rib.
4. Prepare the mop sauce by mixing the soy sauce, beef stock, and bourbon in a food-safe plastic spray bottle.
5. Arrange the ribs directly on the grill and braise for 2 hours, until an internal temperature of 165^0F is reached. Spray the mop sauce over the rib occasionally for tender perfection.
6. Remove rib from the grill and place on an aluminum foil. Pour remaining mop sauce over the ribs and wrap the foil over the ribs.
7. Transfer foil enclosed rib for direct cooking to the grill grate. Braise the ribs until the Instant read thermometer reads a temperature of 195^0F, about one hour.
8. Remove foil enclosed rib from grill and place on a platter to rest for 15 minutes
9. Take out ribs from foil and serve.

Nutritional value per Servings:

Calories: 591kcal, Carbs: 78g, Fat: 13g, Protein: 8g

Veal Paprikash

Veal Paprikash is a classic Hungarian dish. The veal is cooked in sour cream and vegetables, leaving the roast creamy and savory.

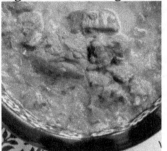

Prep Time and Cooking Time: 1 hour 25 minutes | Serves: 6

Ingredients To Use:

- 3lb Veal, cut into 1-inch piece
- 1 yellow onion, chopped
- 1 tsp cayenne pepper
- 1 small red pepper, finely chopped
- Kosher salt
- 1 cup regular sour cream
- 1 Tsp all-purpose flour
- 1 medium ripe tomato
- 1 Tsp paprika
- 2 Tbsp vegetable oil
- 2 Tbsp butter

Step-by-Step Directions:

1. Preheat wood pellet smoker-grill to 350^{0}F, with the lid closed for about 15 minutes
2. Heat oil and melt butter in a Dutch oven, add the onion and cook until tender, about 3 minutes.
3. Add veal, and then season onion with paprika and cayenne pepper. Cover the lid of the Dutch oven and allow the meat to cook for about 10 minutes.
4. Add tomato, bell pepper, and season with salt. Stir and leave to cook for 45 minutes, until tender.
5. Combine the flour and sour cream in a small bowl. Stir in the flour mixture into the Dutch oven and cook for another 10 minutes.
6. Remove pot from the cooking grid and enjoy the dish.

Nutritional value per servings:

Calories: 400kcal, Carbs: 39g, Fat: 10g, Protein: 38g

Red Wine Beef Stew

Cooked until succulent, chuck roast loaded with carrots, potatoes, and beef is always a hit when braised with rich red wine.

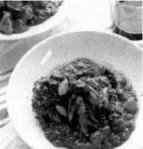

Prep Time and Cooking Time: 3 hours 30 minutes | Serves: 8

Ingredients To Use:

- 1-1/2 tsp kosher salt
- 4lb chuck roast, cut into 2-inch pieces
- 1 Tsp ground black pepper
- 1/4 cup tomato paste
- 1 Tsp olive oil
- 2 cups dry red wine
- 2 bay leaves
- 4 spring's fresh thyme
- 2 lb carrots, peeled and chopped
- 1lb red potatoes, cut into half
- 4 cups chicken broth
- 3 Tsp all-purpose flour

Step-by-Step Directions:

1. Preheat wood pellet smoker-grill to 325°F, with the lid closed for about 15 minutes
2. Place meat in a bowl and sprinkle in salt, pepper, and flour. Toss together until meat is adequately seasoned.
3. Heat oil in a cast-iron Dutch oven and cook the meat at *Medium* for about 8 minutes, until brown.
4. Remove meat and place on a plate. Add wine, broth, tomato paste, thyme, bay leaves, and 1/4 of carrots into the Dutch oven and bring to a boil. Transfer meat to Dutch oven and place on the grill grate for direct cooking. Cook meat for about 2 hours.
5. Remove cooked vegetables from Dutch oven and add remaining carrots and potatoes. Cook until meat is fork-tender, about 1 hour.
6. Serve.

Nutritional value per servings:

Calories: 402kcal, Carbs: 17.3g, Fat: 15.4g, Protein: 35.5g

Chapter 6: Baking Recipes

Banana Walnut bread

This recipe is quick and easy to make. The natural flavor of the banana enhances the delicious taste of the bread.

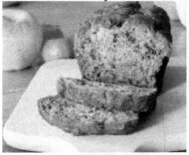

Prep Time and Cooking time: 1 hour 15 minutes / Serves: 1

Ingredients To Use:

- 2-1/2 cup of all-purpose flour
- 1 cup of sugar
- 2 eggs
- 1 cup ripe banana, mashed
- 1/4 cup whole milk
- 1/4 cup walnut, finely chopped
- 1 tsp salt
- 3 Tbsp of Vegetable oil
- 3 tsp baking powder

Step-by-Step Directions:

1. Set the wood pellet smoker-grill for indirect cooking at 350∘F.
2. Combine all the ingredients in a large bowl. Using a mixer (electric or manual), mix the ingredients. Grease and flour the loaf pan. Pour the mixture into the loaf pan.
3. Transfer loaf pan to the grill and cover with steel construction. Bake for 60-75 minutes. Remove and allow to cool.

Nutritional value per serving:

Calories: 548kcal, Carbs: 69g, Fat: 36g, Protein: 14g

Peach Blueberry Cobbler

Blueberry cobbler is an excellent dessert for any meal. It's quick and delicious and tastes even better with vanilla ice-cream at the side.

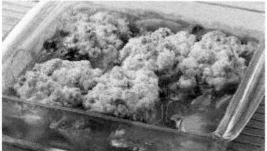

Prep Time and Cooking time: 1hour15 minutesutes / Serves: 4

Ingredients To Use:

- 2 cups of peaches, peeled and sliced
- 1 cup of fresh blueberries
- 1 cup of all-purpose flour
- 1 cup of milk
- 1/2 cup of melted butter, salted
- 2 tsp Baking powder
- 1-1/2 cup sugar
- 1/2 tsp salt
- 1/2 tsp vanilla extract

Step-by-Step Directions:

1. Set the wood pellet smoker-grill to indirect cooking at 375∘F
2. In a bowl, add blueberry, peaches, and ¾ cup sugar. Stir the mixture until the blueberry is coated. Set aside.
3. In another bowl, combine the other ingredients with the remaining sugar and mix well. Be careful not to over stir the mixture.
4. Pour into the baking dish, add the blueberry-peach mixture on top. Do not stir.
5. Transfer baking pan to the grill and cover with steel construction. Bake for 45-60 minutes, remove and allow to rest before serving.

Nutritional value per serving:

Calories: 474kcal, Carbs: 41g, Fat: 25g, Protein: 21g

Baked Wild Sockeye Salmon

Sockeye salmon has a unique, rich flavor. This recipe produces a tender, juicy and flaky salmon. Easy to prepare as it requires a few steps.

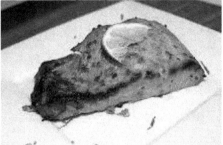

Prep Time and Cooking time: 45 minutes / Serves: 6

Ingredients To Use:

- 6 sockeye salmon fillets
- 3/4 tsp Old bay seasoning
- 1/2 tsp Seafood seasoning.

Step-by-Step Directions:

1. Set the wood pellet smoker-grill to indirect cooking at 400°F
2. Rinse the fillet and pat dry with a paper towel. Add the seasoning, then rub all over the fillets.
3. Arrange fillets in a baking dish with the skin facing down, then transfer the dish to the cooking grid. Cover grill and bake for 15-20 minutes or until fillets begin to flake.
4. Serve.

Nutritional value per serving:

Calories: 294kcal, Carbs: 10g, Fat:1g, Protein: 26g

Pizza dough roll

Pizza dough roll is hot, fresh, and easy to prepare. It can be taken with any meal, but it tastes better with a sauce at the side.

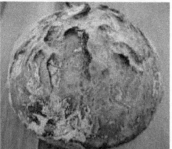

Prep Time and Cooking time: 1hour 15 minutes / Serves: 6

Ingredients To Use:

- 1 tsp Yeast
- 1 cup of warm water
- 2-1/2 cups of all-purpose flour
- 1 tsp Kosher salt
- Tbsp Virgin olive oil
- 1 tsp Sugar

Step-by-Step Directions:

1. Set the wood pellet smoker-grill to indirect cooking at 400°F
2. Combine all your ingredients and mix until the mixture is sticky and has a shaggy texture. Knead the dough for 3-5 minutes, then set aside and cover. Keep for 1 hour at room temperature or until it doubles in size.
3. Divide the dough into six equal parts and roll into a ball using a floured hand. Cover the baking pan with a parchment paper, place the roll on it, then cover and allow to rise for 30 minutes. Transfer the baking pan to the cooking grid, then cover.
4. Bake for 15-20min or until the rolls are golden brown. Allow to cool before serving.

Nutritional value per serving:

Calories: 506kcal, Carbs: 46g, Fat:251g, Protein: 10.1g

Twice-Baked Spaghetti Squash

Spaghetti squash is a versatile side dish. It can also be used as a substitute for pasta when you are on a diet.

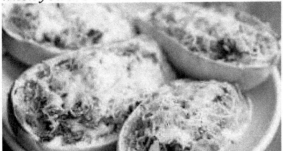

Prep Time and Cooking time:1 hour 15 minutes / Serves: 2

Ingredients To Use:

- 1 medium spaghetti squash
- 1/2 cup of parmesan cheese (grated and divided)
- 1/2 cup of mozzarella cheese (shredded and divided)
- 1 tsp Salt
- Tbsp Extra-virgin olive oil
- 1/2 tsp Pepper

Step-by-Step Directions:

1. Set the wood pellet smoker-grill to indirect cooking at 375∘F
2. Using a knife, cut the squash into half lengthwise and remove the seed and pulp. Rub the inside of the squash with olive oil, salt, and pepper. Place on the hot grill with the open part facing up and bake for 45 minutes or until the squash can be easily pierced with a fork. Remove and allow to cool.
3. Place on a cutting board. Using a fork, scrape across the surface in a lengthwise direction to remove the flesh-in strand (to look like spaghetti). Transfer to a bowl, add parmesan and mozzarella cheese, then stir well. Stuff back into the shell, sprinkle cheese on the toppings.
4. Increase the pellet smoker-grill to 425∘F, place the stuffed squash on the hot grill and bake for 15 minutes or until cheese starts to brown.
5. Remove and allow to cool, serve.

Nutritional value per serving:

Calories: 294kcal, Carbs: 10.1g, Fat:12g, Protein: 16g

Take and Bake Pepperoni Pizza

This is one of the easiest ways to prepare pizza without going through the pains of making the bread. You also get to eat it fresh from the oven.

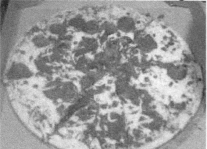

Prep Time and Cooking time: 15 minutes / Serves: 4

Ingredients To Use:

● Take and bake pizza bread
● Pepperoni toppings of your choice

Step-by-Step Directions:

1. Set the wood pellet smoker-grill to indirect cooking at 400∘F
2. If refrigerated, remove pizza bread from the refrigerator 20-30 minutes before baking. Add the toppings and place the bread directly on the cooking grates for a crispier crust.
3. Bake for 10-15 minutes. Remove pizza with a pizza paddle, and allow to cool before cutting into sclices and serving.

Nutritional value per serving:

Calories: 324kcal, Carbs: 31.2g, Fat: 10g, Protein: 14g

Classic Apple Pie

Apple pie is not only one of the best desserts, it can also serve as an excellent entrée for any meal.

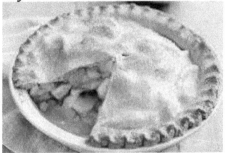

Prep Time and Cooking time: 2 hours / Serves: 8

Ingredients To Use:

- 2 Tbsp all-purpose flour
- 2 pie dough rounds
- 6 cups of apple, peeled and sliced
- 1 Tbsp lemon juice
- 3/4 cup of sugar
- 1/4 tsp powdered nutmeg
- 1/2 tsp powdered cinnamon
- 1/2 tsp salt

Step-by-Step Directions:

1. Set the wood pellet smoker-grill to indirect cooking at 425°F
2. In a large bowl, combine all your ingredients (except for the pie dough) and mix well. Gently press one of the pie dough unto a 10-inch pie dough plate. Make sure it is firm and covers the sides.
3. Pour in your apple mixture. Cover the filling with the second pie dough, gently clip the two doughs together. Make a crosshatch slit on the top with a knife—transfer dough plate to the cooking grid.
4. Bake for 45-60 minutes or until the crust browns. Allow to cool for 1 hour before serving.

Nutritional value per serving:

Calories: 542kcal, Carbs: 41g, Fat: 20g, Protein: 10g

Crusty Artisan Dough Bread

This recipe is great for making a moist, chewy, and crusty bread.

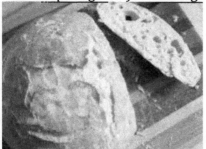

Prep Time and Cooking time: 2 hours / Serves: 6

Ingredients To Use:

- 3 cups all-purpose flour
- 1/2 tsp Yeast
- 1-1/2 cups of warm water
- 1-1/2 tsp salt

Step-by-Step Directions:

1. In a large bowl, combine all your ingredients and mix until it is sticky and has a shaggy texture. Cover with plastic wrap and allow to rest for 12 hours
2. After 12 hours, set the wood pellet smoker-grill to indirect cooking at 425◦F, using any pellet. Preheat the Dutch oven.
3. Transfer prepared mixture to a dry, floured surface and mold into a ball. Open the Dutch oven and place the dough in the middle—cover and bake for 30 minutes.
4. Remove the lid and bake for an additional 20 minutes.
5. Remove and allow to cool.

Nutritional value per serving:

Calories: 462kcal, Carbs: 41g, Fat: 18g, Protein: 5g

Red Chile and Lime Shortbread Cookies

This is a traditional cookie recipe. Red Chile gives the cookie just the right amount of heat.

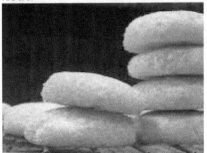

Prep Time and Cooking time: 30 minutes / Serves: 8

Ingredients To Use:

- 2 tsp lime zest
- 8 Tbsp unsalted butter
- 1 cup of all-purpose flour
- 1/2 tsp Salt
- 1 tsp Red Chile rub
- 1/4 cup of sugar

Step-by-Step Directions:

1. Set the wood pellet smoker-grill to indirect cooking at 300∘F
2. In a large bowl, combine all the ingredients (except flour). Mix thoroughly until the butter is creamy but not smooth. Gradually add the flour until it forms a ball.
3. Transfer the dough onto a floured surface, roll until about 1/4-inches thick. Cut into eight equal parts, but do not cut through.
4. Arrange in a cake pan, bake for 10 minutes. Allow to cool before serving.

Nutritional value per serving:

Calories: 478kcal, Carbs: 46g, Fat: 8g, Protein: 2g

Kahluá Coffee Brownies

This is a combination of three different types of chocolate baked into brownies and topped with a rich coffee liqueur.

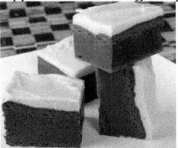

Prep Time and Cooking time: 60 minutes / Serves: 12

Ingredients To Use:

- 4 oz. pure chocolate, unsweetened
- 1 cup of white chocolate chip
- 1 cup of bittersweet chocolate chip
- 4 eggs
- 1/8 Tsp of salt
- Tbsp instant coffee
- 1-1/2 cup all-purpose flour
- cups of sugar
- 1 cup unsalted butter

Step-by-Step Directions:

1. Set the wood pellet smoker-grill to indirect cooking at 350∘F
2. Place a small pot on the cooking grid, then add the butter and coffee. Stir until it melts completely. Remove the pot from heat and stir in the unsweetened chocolate, stir until it is smooth. Add the eggs one at a time, mix well. While still mixing, add the sugar, flour, and salt. Gently fold the white chocolate and bittersweet chocolate into the mixture.
3. Pour the mixture into a baking pan and bake on the grates for 20 minutes or until a toothpick comes out clean.
4. Remove and allow to cool.

Nutritional value per serving:

Calories: 589kcal, Carbs: 60g, Fat: 42g, Protein: 24g

Twice- Baked potatoes with Smoked Gouda and grilled scallions

This recipe is rich and creamy; the smoked gouda adds a unique flavor to it—the perfect meal for a dinner party.

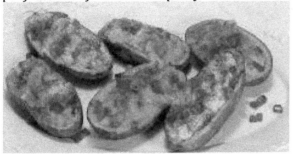

Prep Time and Cooking time: 1hours 15 minutes / Serves: 6

Ingredients To Use:

- 3 large potatoes
- 8 TbspUnsalted butter
- Tbsp Of barbeque rub
- 1-1/2 cup of smoked gouda cheese (grated)
- 1/4 cup of extra-virgin olive oil
- 3/4 cup heavy cream
- Salt and pepper to taste
- 1/4 cup chopped scallions

Step-by-Step Directions:

1. Set the wood pellet smoker-grill to indirect cooking at 400°F
2. Brush the potatoes with olive oil, make incisions with fork and season with salt. Wrap with aluminum foil paper and bake on grill grates for 30 minutes per side. Transfer to a rimmed sheet and allow to cool.
3. Cut the potatoes lengthwise, scoop out the flesh into a bowl. Add butter and 1 cup of cheese. Set aside. Place a small pot over low-medium heat, add cream, then heat for 1 minute. Add the scallions and the barbeque rub and mix well
4. Add the scallion mixture to the potatoes and cheese in the bowl, combine until it is evenly mixed. Scoop the mixture back into the potato shell and top with cheese.
5. Bake for 5 minutes or until the cheese melts.

Nutritional value per serving:

Calories: 276kcal, Carbs: 28g, Fat: 14.5g, Protein: 3g

Chocolate Pecan Bourbon Pie

Pecan pie is a traditional pie recipe that combines the flavor of bourbon and chocolate. A good dessert to top your meal during the holidays.

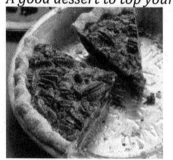

Prep Time and Cooking time: 60 minutes / Serves: 6

Ingredients To Use:

- 1/4 cup bourbon
- 1 cup semisweet chocolate chips
- 1 cup of dark corn syrup
- Tbsp of melted unsalted butter
- 3 large egg (beaten)
- 1 cup of pecan (chopped)
- 1 cup of brown sugar
- 1 pie shell

Step-by-Step Directions:

1. Set the wood pellet smoker-grill to indirect cooking at 400°F
2. In a bowl, combine the corn syrup, egg, butter, sugar, and bourbon. Then add the chocolate chips and mix well. Pour the filling into the pie shell.
3. Place the pie plates on the grid and bake for 45 minutes or until fillings turn brown.
4. Remove and allow to cool. Refrigerate or serve.

Nutritional value per serving:

Calories: 560kcal, Carbs: 38g, Fat: 23.5g, Protein: 10g

Chapter 7: Searing Recipe

Pan-Seared Lamb Chops

This seared lamb chops recipe is perfect for a dinner meal. And it tastes better with mascarpone sauce and red wine.

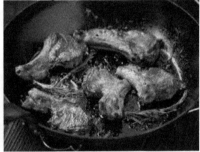

Prep Time and Cooking time: 40 minutes / Serves: 6

Ingredients To Use:

- 12 fresh lamb chops
- 2 Tbsp Olive oil
- 1/2 Tbsp Pepper
- 1/2 Tbsp Salt.

Step-by-Step Directions:

1. Preheat the wood pellet smoker-grill for direct cooking at 300°F using any pellet.
2. Rinse the lamb chops and pat dry with a paper towel, season with salt and pepper.
3. Grill both sides of lamb chops for 20 minutes, then increase the temperature of the grill to *High.*
4. Place an iron skillet over the cooking grid, add olive oil, and sear the chops for 3 minutes per side or until it is golden brown.
5. Place on the baking sheet and roast for 10 minutes or until the internal temperature is 125°F.

Nutritional value per serving:

Calories: 361kcal, Carbs: 14g, Fat: 21g, Protein: 48g

Pan-Seared Lamb Loins with Horseradish Potato Gratin

Lamb loins are especially delicious when pan-seared. Spicy horseradish and potatoes make a tasty side dish for the lamb.

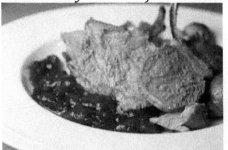

Prep Time and Cooking time: 2hours / Serves: 6

Ingredients To Use:

- 2 lamb loins
- 2 Tbsp Olive oil
- 1-1/2 Tbsp Pepper
- 1-1/2 Tbsp Salt.
- 2 Tbsp prepared horseradish
- Tbsp Unsalted butter
- 1/2 cup of crumbled goat cheese
- 1 cup of whipped cream
- potatoes, peeled and sliced
- 1/2 cup of parmesan cheese

Step-by-Step Directions:

1. Preheat the wood pellet smoker-grill for direct cooking at 300°F using any pellet.
2. Rinse the lamb chops and pat dry with a paper towel, season with salt and pepper.
3. Grill the lamb loins for 15 minutes, then set the temperature of the grill to *High*
4. Place an iron skillet on the cooking grid, add olive oil, then sear the lamb for 10 minutes until brown on all sides. Perform this action carefully to prevent the lamb from burning; it will develop a bitter taste.
5. Allow it to rest before slicing.
6. Grease a large baking dish with butter. In a large bowl, combine the cream, parmesan cheese, goat cheese, horseradish, salt, and pepper. Whisk together and drop the sliced potatoes into the mixture.

7. Arrange the potatoes in the baking dish and cover with plastic wrap, then add a layer of aluminum foil and bake for 1 hour. Remove the cover and bake for another 30 minutes.
8. Serve with the lamb.

Nutritional value per serving:

Calories: 467kcal, Carbs: 28.9g, Fat: 25g, Protein: 42.6g

Reverse-Seared Halibut

Halibuts have a unique taste and flavor. This recipe is another excellent way of preparing halibut fillets.

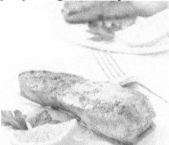

Prep Time and Cooking time: 50 minutes / Serves: 4

Ingredients To Use:

- halibut fillet (skin removed)
- 1 tsp of salt
- 1 tsp grounded black pepper
- 1 tsp of dried basil
- 1 tbsp lemon juice
- Pinch of chopped parsley
- tbsps olive oil.

Step-by-Step Directions:

1. Preheat the wood pellet smoker-grill for direct cooking at 300◦F.
2. In a large bowl, add the fillets, salt, basil, olive oil, salt, pepper, and lemon juice. Cover and refrigerate for 30 minutes.
3. Grill the halibut for 30 minutes, then set aside.
4. Increase the temperature to 450◦F and allow the temperature of the grill to rise.
5. Sear halibut for 3 minutes per side. Remove and garnish with parsley.

Nutritional value per serving:

Calories: 517kcal, Carbs: 2g, Fat: 23g, Protein: 37g

Salt-Seared Calf Liver and Beacon

One bite of this delicious recipe will ignite your taste bud. Searing the liver on a salt block with a dash of beacon creates a unique taste

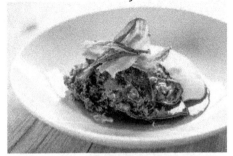

Prep Time and Cooking time: 30 minutes / Serves: 2

Ingredients To Use:

- 1 (8-inch) square salt block
- Tbsp Sherry vinegar
- Tbsp Parsley, fresh and finely chopped
- 1 piece of bacon, thick and quartered
- 12 oz. Calf liver
- Salt and pepper to taste

Step-by-Step Directions:

1. Preheat the wood pellet smoker-grill for direct cooking at 350∘F using any pellet.
2. Place the salt block on the pellet smoker-grill and heat for 10 minutes, increase the temperature to 450∘F (*High*), and heat for another 10 minutes. While heating the salt block, season the liver with salt and pepper.
3. Place the bacon on the salt block and heat until crisp, mop excess fat dripping from the bacon. Remove and allow to cool. Place the liver on the salt block and sear for 2 minutes per side.
4. Transfer to a plate, add the beacon, and drizzle with vinegar. Sprinkle the parsley.

Nutritional value per serving:

Calories: 354kcal, Carbs: 27.8g, Fat: 21.5g, Protein: 36.3g

Pan-seared Pork Tenderloin with Apple Mashed Potatoes

The combination of pork, applesauce, and mashed potatoes gives a surprisingly tang flavor. The meat is enriched with the sauce, which enhances the flavor.

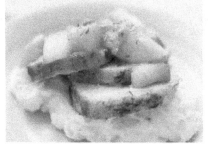

Prep Time and Cooking time: 20 minutes / Serves: 6

Ingredients To Use:

- 2 pork tenderloin
- medium potatoes (peeled and sliced)
- 3 Tbsp unsalted butter
- 1/2 cup of heavy cream
- 2 Tbsp Olive oil
- 1-1/2 Tbsp Pepper
- 1-1/2 Tbsp Salt.
- 2 apple (cored and sliced)

Step-by-Step Directions:

1. Preheat the wood pellet smoker-grill for direct cooking at 300°F using any pellet.
2. Season the pork with salt and pepper, then roast meat for 20 minutes.
3. Increase the temperature of the grill to *High,* then place an iron skillet on the grates, and add 1 Tbsp butter and oil. Cook until the butter becomes brown, make sure it does not burn.
4. Place the tenderloin and cook for 4 minutes per side or until it is brown, transfer to a baking sheet and bake for 10 minutes.
5. Rearrange the grill for indirect cooking at 300°F
6. Place a pot over the cooking grid and fill it with water. Add potatoes and allow to boil, reduce the heat and simmer for 8 minutes or until soft. Drain the water
7. Pour the potatoes into a food processor, add cream and butter. Puree the mixture, add the apples and puree until they are finely chopped. Season with salt and pepper and serve with the pork.

Nutritional value per serving:

Calories: 477kcal, Carbs: 26.9g, Fat: 24.5g, Protein: 46.5g

Pan-seared Ribeye Steak with Parsley Potatoes

The heat gives this ribeye recipe a crusty coating. It is moist, tender, and melts in the mouth.

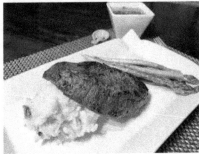

Prep Time and Cooking time: 60 minutes / Serves: 6

Ingredients To Use:

- 2 pork tenderloin
- medium potatoes (peeled and sliced)
- 3 tbsps extra-virgin olive oil
- 2 Tbsp Fresh parsley (chopped)
- Salt and pepper to taste.

Step-by-Step Directions:

1. Preheat the wood pellet smoker-grill for direct cooking at 300◦F using any pellets
2. Rinse the meat and pat dry, then season with salt and pepper.
3. Grill pork for 20 minutes, then set aside and increase the temperature of the grill to *High.*
4. Place an iron skillet on grill grates, add the oil and heat for 1 minute. Sear the meat for 3 minutes per side or until brown. Allow it to rest before serving.
5. Rearrange the grill for indirect cooking at 300◦F
6. Place a pot on grates and fill with water, add the potatoes and allow to boil, reduce the heat and simmer for 15 minutes or until the potatoes become soft. Drain the water. Transfer to a bowl, add parsley, and olive oil.
7. Serve with pork.

Nutritional value per serving:

Calories: 354kcal, Carbs: 27.8g, Fat: 21.5g, Protein: 36g

Reverse-Seared Tilapia

This recipe is delicious and easy to prepare. Perfect for a weekday dinner and better enjoyed with wine.

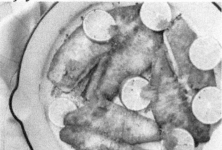

Prep Time and Cooking time: 20 minutes / Serves: 4

Ingredients To Use:

- tilapia fillets
- 2 Tbsp melted butter (unsalted)
- 1/2 cup of all-purpose flour
- Salt and pepper to taste

Step-by-Step Directions:

1. Preheat the wood pellet smoker-grill for direct cooking at 350°F using any pellet
2. Rinse the fillets and pat dry with a paper towel. Season with salt and pepper, coat with the flour.
3. Transfer Tilapia fillets to cooking grate and grill for 20 minutes or until internal temperature measure 150°F. Then set fillets aside and increase the temperature of the grill to 450°F
4. Sear the tilapia for 4 minutes per side or until it flakes. Brush melted butter on the tilapia.
5. Serve.

Nutritional value per serving:

Calories: 295kcal, Carbs: 11.2g, Fat: 16g, Protein: 24.6g

Salt-Seared Prawn

Searing prawns with a salt block will have you licking your fingers. The salt and spices combine to bring out a tasty and delicious prawn.

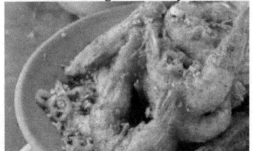

Prep Time and Cooking time: 1 hour 20 minutes / Serves: 4

Ingredients To Use:

- 2 lb. Prawns, head intact
- 2 lb. Salt rock
- 1 lime, cut into 8 wedges
- Pinch of crushed red pepper flakes
- 12 black peppercorn, smashed
- 4-star anise pod, pieced
- cinnamon stick, broken to pieces

Step-by-Step Directions:

1. Preheat the wood pellet smoker-grill for indirect cooking at 300◦F using any pellet.
2. Mix the cinnamon, peppercorns, pepper flakes, anise, then bake for 40 minutes.
3. Place the salt block on the pellet smoker-grill and heat for 10 minutes, then increase the temperature to 450◦F (*High*), and heat for another 10 minutes.
4. Sear the prawn for 4 minutes per side. Serve the prawn with the lime wedges.

Nutritional value per serving:

Calories: 254kcal, Carbs: 6g, Fat: 2g, Protein: 10g

Salt-Seared Kobe Beef with Tarragon Shallot Butter

Traeger grilled beef is typically delicious, but when grilled on a salt block, it tastes extraordinary.

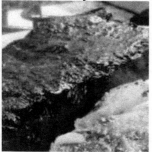

Prep Time and Cooking time: 40 minutes / Serves: 4

Ingredients To Use:

- 1 (8-inch) square salt block
- 3 Tbsp Unsalted butter
- 2 finely chopped shallot
- 12 oz. Kobe beef, boneless, trimmed, then boiled
- Grounded black pepper to taste
- 1/4 cup of dry vermouth
- Finely chopped tarragon leaves (1 sprig)

Step-by-Step Directions:

1. Preheat the wood pellet smoker-grill for direct cooking at 400◦F using any pellet
2. Heat the salt block on the smoker-grill for 10 minutes, increase the temperature to 450◦F (High), and heat for another 10 minutes. While the salt is heating, transfer your beef to a freezer for 10-15 minutes. Do not allow to freeze.
3. Place a medium skillet on the cooking grate, then add the vermouth and shallot. Stir occasionally to prevent the shallot from boiling dry. Boil until 1 tbsp of shallot remains in the skillet, stir in the pepper and tarragon. Allow to cool and mix with butter.
4. Remove the beef and slice to about 1/4 -inch-thickness. Sear for 5 minutes per side on the salt block. Serve with shallot-tarragon butter.

Nutritional value per serving:

Calories: 342kcal, Carbs: 16g, Fat: 12g, Protein: 32g

Seared Venison Chops with Marsala

Venison is rich in flavor, juicy, and tender like pork. It can be eaten with wine sauce and rice.

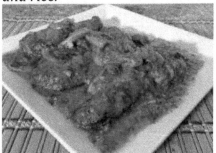

Prep Time and Cooking time: 1 hour 10 minutes / Serves: 6

Ingredients To Use:

- 1 cup marsala wine
- Venison chops
- 3 Tbsp unsalted butter
- 2 Tbsp olive oil
- 1 cup of beef stock
- 1 tsp fresh sage, finely chopped
- 1 cup of beef stock
- Salt and pepper to taste
- peeled shallot

Step-by-Step Directions:

1. Set the wood pellet smoker-grill to direct cooking at 300∘F
2. Rinse the venison and pat dry with a paper towel. Season with salt and pepper.
3. Grill both sides of venison for 30 minutes, then set aside and increase the temperature of the grill to *High.*
4. Place a skillet over cooking grates, add oil and sear venison for 4 minutes per side. Set aside.
5. Place a small pot over cooking grates, melt 1 tbsp of butter and sauté the shallot for 5 minutes, or until they are brown.
6. Add the stock, marsala, and sage and allow it to simmer for 15-20 minutes. Add the remaining butter, season with salt and pepper.
7. Serve with the venison.

Nutritional value per serving:

Calories: 345kcal, Carbs: 24g, Fat: 23.5g, Protein: 45g

Chapter 8: Marinade, Rub and Sauce

Texas-Style Brisket Rub

This rub is a combination of different spices that will give your brisket a sweet and unique taste. Apply on the brisket and allow to sit for 3-4hours or refrigerate overnight.

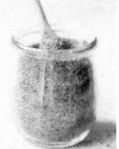

Prep Time and Cooking time: 15 minutes / Serves: 1

Ingredients To Use:

- 2 tsp Sugar
- 2 Tbsp Kosher salt
- 2 tsp Chilli powder
- 2 Tbsp Black pepper
- Tbsp Cayenne pepper
- Tbsp Powdered garlic
- tsp Grounded cumin
- 2 Tbsp Powdered onion
- 1/4 cup paprika, smoked

Step-by-Step Directions:

1. Mix all the ingredients in a small bowl until it is well blended.
2. Transfer to an airtight jar or container. Store in a cool place.

Nutritional value per serving:

Calories: 18kcal, Carbs: 2g, Fat: 1g, Protein: 0.6g

Pork Dry Rub

This rub can be used in the preparation of different pork recipes. The amount used for your food depends on your taste.

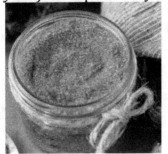

Prep Time and Cooking time: 15 minutes / Serves: 1 cup

Ingredients To Use:

- Tbsp Kosher salt
- 2 Tbsp Powered onions
- Tbsp Cayenne pepper
- 1tsp Dried mustard
- 1/4 cup brown sugar
- Tbsp Powdered garlic
- Tbsp Powdered chili pepper
- 1/4 cup smoked paprika
- 2 Tbsp Black pepper

Step-by-Step Directions:

1. Combine all the ingredients in a small bowl.
2. Transfer to an airtight jar or container.
3. Keep stored in a cool, dry place.

Nutritional value per serving:

Calories: 16kcal, Carbs: 3g, Fat:0.9g, Protein: 0.8g

Texas Barbeque Rub

This rub can be used for beef, poultry, pork, and other types of meat and vegetables. It can either be rubbed on the surface of food and smoked immediately or rubbed on food then refrigerated to allow marinate

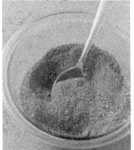

Prep Time and Cooking time: 15 minutes / Serves: 1/2 cup

Ingredients To Use:

- 1 tsp Sugar
- Tbsp Seasoned salt
- Tbsp Black pepper
- tsp Chilli powder
- Tbsp Powdered onions
- Tbsp Smoked paprika
- 1 tsp Sugar
- Tbsp Powdered garlic

Step-by-Step Directions:

1. Pour all the ingredients into a small bowl and mix thoroughly.
2. Keep stored in an airtight jar or container.

Nutritional value per serving:

Calories: 22kcal, Carbs: 2g, Fat: 0.2g, Protein: 0.6g

Barbeque Sauce

This is a classic sauce with the right amount of sweetness and spice. If you are interested in a simple sauce for your barbecue, this is perfect.

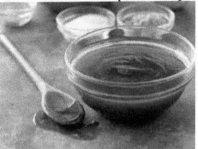

Prep Time and Cooking time: 15 minutes / Serves: 2 cups

Ingredients To Use:

- 1/4 cup of water
- 1/4 cup red wine vinegar
- Tbsp Worcestershire sauce
- 1 tsp Paprika
- 1 tsp Salt
- Tbsp Dried mustard
- 1 tsp black pepper
- 1 cup ketchup
- 1 cup brown sugar

Step-by-Step Directions:

1. Pour all the ingredients into a food processor, one after the other.
2. Process until they are evenly mixed.
3. Transfer sauce to a close lid jar. Store in the refridgerator.

Nutritional value per serving:

Calories: 43kcal, Carbs: 10g Fat: 0.3g, Protein: 0.9g

Steak Sauce

This sauce brings out the unique flavor and texture in steaks. The presence of raspberry in this recipe adds a twist to the flavor.

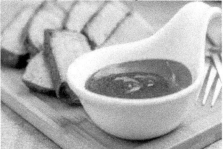

Prep Time and Cooking time: 25 minutes / Serves: ½ cup

Ingredients To Use:

- Tbsp Malt vinegar
- 1/2 tsp Salt
- 1/2 tsp black pepper
- Tbsp Tomato sauce
- 2 Tbsp brown sugar
- 1 tsp hot pepper sauce
- 2 Tbsp Worcestershire sauce
- 2 Tbsp Raspberry jam.

Step-by-Step Directions:

1. Preheat your grill for indirect cooking at 150°F
2. Place a saucepan over grates, add all your ingredients, and allow to boil.
3. Reduce the temperature to *Smoke* and allow the sauce to simmer for 10 minutes or until sauce is thick.

Nutritional value per serving:

Calories: 62.1kcal, Carbs: 15.9g Fat: 0.3g, Protein:0.1g

Bourbon Whiskey Sauce

Bourbon whiskey sauce is a nice and tasty barbecue sauce recipe. It contains lots of spices and ingredients. For better taste, refrigerate a day or two before use.

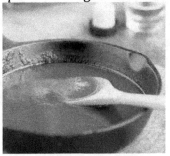

Prep Time and Cooking time: 45 minutes / Serves: 3cup

Ingredients To Use:

- cups ketchup
- 1/4 cup Worcestershire sauce
- 3/4 cup bourbon whiskey
- 1/3 cup apple cider vinegar
- 1/2 onions, minced
- 1/4 cup of tomato paste
- cloves of garlic, minced
- 1/2 tsp Black pepper
- 1/2 cup brown sugar
- 1/2 Tbsp Salt
- Hot pepper sauce to taste
- Tbsp Liquid smoke flavoring

Step-by-Step Directions:

1. Preheat your grill for indirect cooking at 150°F
2. Place a saucepan over grates, then add the whiskey, garlic, and onions.
3. Simmer until the onion is translucent. Then add the other ingredients and adjust the temperature to *Smoke*. Simmer for 20 minutes. For a smooth sauce, sieve.

Nutritional value per serving:

Calories: 107kcal, Carbs:16.6g Fat: 1.8g, Protein:0.8g

Chicken Marinade

This marinade is of Asian origins; it makes your chicken juicy and succulent. It brings out the best taste in your chicken.

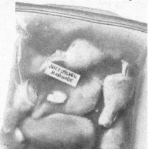

Prep Time and Cooking time: 35 minutes / Serves: 3 cups

Ingredients To Use:

- halved chicken breast (bone and skin removed)
- Tbsp Spicy brown mustard
- 2/3 cup of soy sauce
- tsp Powdered garlic
- 2 Tbsp Liquid smoke flavoring
- 2/3 cup extra virgin olive oil
- 2/3 cup lemon juice
- 2 tsp Black pepper

Step-by-Step Directions:

1. Mix all the ingredients in a large bowl.
2. Pour the chicken into the bowl and allow it to marinate for about 3-4hours in the refrigerator. Remove the chicken, then smoke, grill, or roast the chicken.

Nutritional value per serving:

Calories: 507kcal, Carbs:46.6g Fat: 41.8g, Protein: 28g

Carne Asada Marinade

This marinade contains simple spices that bring out the unique flavor of your meat. Easy to prepare.

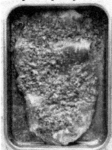

Prep Time and Cooking time: 2hours / Serves: 5 cups

Ingredients To Use:

- cloves garlic, chopped
- tsp Lemon juice
- 1/2 cup extra virgin olive oil
- 1/2 tsp Salt
- 1/2 tsp Pepper

Step-by-Step Directions:

1. Mix all your ingredients in a bowl.
2. Pour the beef into the bowl and allow to marinate for 2-3hours before grilling.

Nutritional value per serving:

Calories: 465kcal, Carbs: 26g Fat: 15g, Protein: 28g

Grapefruit Juice Marinade

This marinade gives your chicken a nice juicy and tasty oriental flavor. It is spicy with the right amount of sweetness.

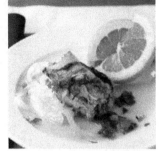

Prep Time and Cooking time: 1hours 10 minutes / Serves: 3 cups

Ingredients To Use:

- 1/2 reduced-sodium soy sauce
- cups grapefruit juice, unsweetened
- 1-1/2 lb. Chicken, bone and skin removed
- 1/4 brown sugar

Step-by-Step Directions:

1. Thoroughly mix all your ingredients in a large bowl.
2. Add the chicken and allow it to marinate for 2-3 hours before grilling.

Nutritional value per serving:

Calories: 489kcal, Carbs: 21.3g Fat: 12g, Protein: 24g

Steak Marinade

This marinade is straightforward to prepare. It is a blend of different spice and sauce to give a sweet and tasty flavor.

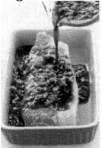

Prep Time and Cooking time: 15 minutes / Serves: 2cups

Ingredients To Use:

- Tbsp Worcestershire sauce
- Tbsp Red wine vinegar
- 1/2 cup barbeque sauce
- Tbsp soy sauce
- 1/4 cup steak sauce
- 1 clove garlic (minced)
- 1 tsp Mustard
- Pepper and salt to taste

Step-by-Step Directions:

1. Pour all the ingredients in a bowl and mix thoroughly.
2. Use immediately or keep refrigerated.

Nutritional value per serving:

Calories: 303kcal, Carbs: 42g Fat: 10g, Protein:2.4g

Conversion Chart

U.S. Volume Measure	Metric Equivalent
1/8 teaspoon (tsp)	0.5 milliliter
1/4 teaspoon	1 milliliter
1/2 teaspoon	2 milliliters
1 teaspoon	5 milliliters
1/2 tablespoon (Tbsp)	7 milliliters
1 tablespoon (3 tsp)	15 milliliters
2 tablespoons (1 fluid ounce)	30 milliliters
1/4 cup	60 milliliters
1/3 cup	90 milliliters
1/2 cup (4 fluid ounces)	125 milliliters
2/3 cup	160 milliliters
3/4 cup	180 milliliters
1 cup (8 fluid ounces)	250 milliliters
2 cups	460 milliliters
4 cups	0.95 liter or 950 milliliters
1 quart	1 liter
4 quarts (1 gallon)	3.8 liters

WEIGHT AND LENGTH CONVERSIONS

U.S Weight Measure	Metric Equivalent
1/2 ounce	14 grams
1 ounce	28 grams
2 ounces	57 grams
3 ounces	85 grams
1/4 pound (4 ounces)	113 grams
1/2 pound (8 ounces)	227 grams
3/4 pound (12 ounces)	340 grams
1 pound (16 ounces)	454 grams
2.2 pounds (35.25 ounces)	1 kilogram
Length	**Metric Equivalent**

1/8 inch	3 millimeters
1/4 inch	6 millimeters
1/2 inch	1¼ centimeters
1 inch	2½ centimeters
2 inches	5 centimeters
4 inches	10 centimeters
5 inches	13 centimeters
6 inches	15-1/4 centimeters
12 inches (1 foot)	30 centimeters

OVEN TEMPERATURE CONVERSIONS

Degrees Fahrenheit	Degrees Celsius
200°F	95°C
225°F	110°C
250°F	120°C
275°F	135°C
300°F	150°C
325°F	160°C
350°F	180°C
375°F	190°C
400°F	200°C
425°F	220°C
450°F	230°C
475°F	245°C
600°F	316°C

CPSIA information can be obtained
at www.ICGtesting.com
Printed in the USA
LVHW011916291020
670161LV00004B/327